Therapy Tech

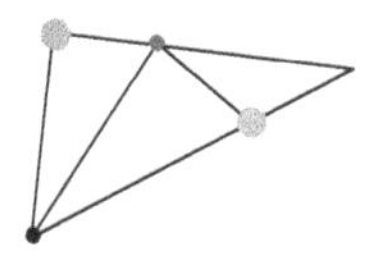

Therapy Tech

The Digital Transformation of Mental Healthcare

Emma Bedor Hiland

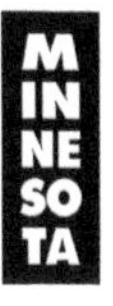

University of Minnesota Press
Minneapolis
London

Published by the University of Minnesota Press
111 Third Avenue South, Suite 290
Minneapolis, MN 55401-2520
http://www.upress.umn.edu

ISBN 978-1-5179-1116-4 (hc)
ISBN 978-1-5179-1117-1 (pb)

Library of Congress record available at https://lccn.loc.gov/2021022897

UMP LSI

For Alex

Contents

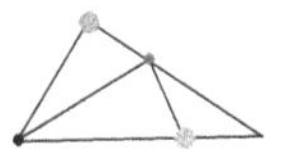

Introduction

Pursuing a Technological Fix

In 2017 the Food and Drug Administration granted approval for the very first medication to include an ingestible sensor: Abilify MyCite. This drug's approval was significant, its advocates believed, because including a tracking tool would encourage prescription medication adherence.[1] Yet the Food and Drug Administration's press release at the time contained a clause that called MyCite's ability to do so into question, noting that "the ability of the product to improve patient compliance with their treatment regimen has not been shown."[2]

Without any actual data to suggest that including a tracking device would increase medication adherence, it should come as no surprise that Abilify MyCite's approval was also met with skepticism and concern. Dr. Paul Applebaum, former president of the American Psychological Association, argued that adding a tracker to an antipsychotic would do nothing to remedy existing reasons people do not take those medications, including negative side effects, a patient's belief that drugs are not needed, or, as is often the case of persons to whom Abilify is prescribed, paranoia.[3] "You would think that, whether in psychiatry or general medicine, drugs for almost any other condition would be a better place to start than a drug for schizophrenia," Applebaum stated.[4]

I begin this book with a discussion of Abilify MyCite's approval because the discourse surrounding its release exemplifies this book's foremost problematic: technologies, in various forms, are believed to be solutions to the United States' ongoing mental health crisis. Estimates suggest that roughly one in five Americans now lives with a mental illness,[5] and other data indicate that

50 percent will experience mental illness at some point during their lifetimes.[6] The United States also continues to be faced with practitioner scarcity[7] and an inability to provide mental healthcare services to geographically remote destinations,[8] and charges such high fees for mental healthcare services that they are often rendered inaccessible for those who need them.[9] Yet the belief that mental health's technologization—that is, its technological transformation—can solve the mental healthcare crisis is unfounded. Just as inserting a tracking device into an antipsychotic does not address the underlying reasons persons already do not take their prescribed medications, the technologies discussed in this book should be similarly understood. They are ineffectual Band-Aids, in no way up to the task of repairing a broken mental healthcare system. Instead of addressing the systemic, structural barriers to accessing and receiving quality mental healthcare in the United States and beyond, we fetishize novel technologies because innovation excites us. Yet prioritizing novelty over efficacy is to our detriment, as we come to forget our initial goal: to fundamentally increase the accessibility of mental healthcare services.

Technological interventions are incapable of solving disparities and inequities which pre-date them, and therefore belief in technology's ability to improve our lives without also addressing structural inequalities is sorely misplaced. Health-related inequities are not merely the result of "glitches," "bugs," or flaws in the design(s) of technologies themselves, problems that (if they did originate in technologies) might be remedied by rewriting code or adjusting algorithms. Rather, these problems result from human activities, behaviors, and systems of belief that have already shaped and molded culture and medicine for hundreds of years. When the domains of technology and medicine intersect, therefore, the likelihood of deeply entrenched discriminatory belief systems and practices manifesting becomes vastly greater. Those who believe that technology is "the key to solving mental healthcare access problems in the twenty-first century,"[10] a position suggested by psychologist Bartley Christopher Frueh, are merely propagating techno-solutionism, disregarding the reality that racism, sexism, classism, and other discriminatory belief systems contributed to the mental healthcare crisis in the first place.

This book should be understood as more than merely a study of those technologies which claim to improve user mental health. This book is also a study of faith in technology and a demonstration of why that faith is misplaced. The question we should be asking is not how might we create technologies capable of solving the mental healthcare crisis, but rather what do mental health technologies reveal about beliefs and practices related to the self, medicine, and culture? This book responds to that query by demonstrating that mental health technologies are an outgrowth of a neoliberal ethos of care, perpetuating hegemonic ideals of individual responsibilization while also demanding their users enact new forms of labor, participate in new types of surveillance, and adopt entrepreneurial attitudes toward their own mental healthiness. These findings also demonstrate, on a practical level, that mental health technologies will fail if ever proffered as solutions to the ongoing mental healthcare crisis. Many are discriminatory in design, unusable for all populations equally, and facilitate the perpetuation of existing disparities related to race, gender, and socioeconomic status.

There is not, and never will be, a technological solution to the mental healthcare crisis. What is true, however, is that mental health technologies—whether ingestible sensors, smartphone applications, or therapeutic chatbots fueled by advances in machine learning and artificial intelligence—are causing vast changes in the realms of medicine, technology, and popular culture. Yet those changes are a matter distinct and separate from improvements in the quality and accessibility of mental healthcare services. Instead they are related to the relationship(s) between culture, technology, health, and medicine, and the ways in which technologies both reflect our beliefs and values while simultaneously shaping them.

My hope is that this book serves as a catalyst for increased critical thinking and conversation about the role of technology in our lives, not only related to how we care for ourselves in matters of mental health, but also what the actual, practical limits of technologies are. To dream of technological solutions is to imagine a better future, but to actually direct vast resources to the development of technologies that are incapable of providing what we need is wasteful. While this book presents these arguments in the context of mental health technologies, it more broadly demonstrates that there will always be disparities between technologies' actual capabilities and our imaginings about what they can accomplish.

Neoliberalism and Mental Health

This book positions mental health technologies as illustrative of the expansion and intensification of a neoliberal ethos, an orientation to individual responsibilization so vast that, today, even mental health is presumably within one's own control. Although matters of the mind were once considered knowable (and by extension treatable) only by those with expertise in the mental health professions, the individuation of responsibility has led to a significant shift wherein we are encouraged to believe that participation in regimes of technologically facilitated practices empower us. In turn, each of us is rendered competent to manage our own mental health.

Neoliberalism as discussed in this book comes from the work of Michel Foucault, and draws attention to the ways that economic principles and rationalities have permeated all domains of culture and life. It is under these conditions that individuals are encouraged—and expected—to care for themselves through privatized, self-directed means as systems of large-scale support (originating from government proper) are reduced.[11] Prior scholarship on the intersections of health and neoliberalism explores an array of phenomena, including how overweight persons are encouraged to win their personal "wars" on obesity,[12] the effects of direct-to-consumer advertising upon audiences,[13] television's metamorphosis into a therapeutic device,[14] how men's magazines encourage readers to self-manage health risks,[15] and much, much more.

Importantly, despite the diminishing role of the State under neoliberalism, power itself is neither reduced nor eliminated. Citizens are still encouraged to act and behave in ways that serve the State's interests even without sovereign powers explicitly directing them to. Foucault describes this process as *governmentality*, in which persons become disposed to act in certain ways rather than compelled.[16] Power still exists and operates, though it does so through dispersed mechanisms and channels. Governmentality, Foucault explains, involves "employing tactics rather than laws, and even of using laws themselves as tactics—to arrange things in such a way that, through a certain number of means, such and such ends may be achieved . . . and the instruments of government, instead of being laws, now come to be a range of multiform tactics."[17]

Consider the following examples of "multiform tactics," to use Foucault's phrase, offered by insurance companies to encourage individuals to manage their health via self-tracking technologies: Oscar gives its members one dollar toward Amazon gift cards when they hit their desired daily step counts,[18] UnitedHealthcare deposits rewards into members' reimbursement accounts for meeting health goals,[19] and one of the benefits of enrolling in John Hancock's Vitality program is that members can save up to 15 percent on their healthcare policies.[20] Yet good citizenship practices, which involve taking responsibility for our health, start long before we choose an insurance plan. Now even educational institutions "encourage" the utilization of technologies in the pursuit of fitness: Oklahoma's Oral Roberts University asks that its students wear FitBits to track their daily steps,[21] and Adidas created devices for students in elementary, middle, and high school to wear that enable physical education teachers to track their activity levels.[22] Despite the absence of explicit, disciplinary force requiring that we utilize these technologies, they nonetheless demonstrate the ways in which technoreliant health practices come to be normalized and encouraged, beginning during childhood. Our compliance is expected, though not mandated.

Inactivity is an established risk factor for a number of chronic illnesses, negative health outcomes and, by extension, increased healthcare costs.[23] It makes sense, therefore, that money-minded insurance companies would want their policy holders to be active and, by extension, healthy. Just as the turn toward fitness-encouraging technologies is motivated by economic rationales, so too is the turn toward technological interventions promoting mental healthiness. Research suggests that depression is on the rise for all populations in the United States,[24] and other findings add that teenagers and young adults are experiencing more mood disorders than ever before.[25] In 2005 depression was estimated to generate a loss of roughly $173.2 billion to the U.S. economy and by 2010 that number ballooned to $210.5 billion.[26] By 2030, it is believed, mental illness will cost the global economy $16 trillion.[27] Yet before we accept at face value that preventative mental health technologies are warranted because of exponential growth in diagnoses of mental illnesses, we should question the veracity of the claim that "more" people are experiencing mental illness than ever before. As cultural studies scholar Nikolas Rose points out, while it is certainly possible that there is "more mental disorder today than in previous times," there are other potential contributing factors to consider:

> We are more aware of mental disorder and better at recognizing it. . . . it is the pharmaceutical companies, in a cynical search for market share, profit and shareholder value, who . . . are distorting our perception and treatment of mental disorder . . . [and] that this arises from a reshaping of our discontents in a psychiatric form—perhaps even a psychiatrization of the human condition itself.[28]

This last hypothesis, of psychiatrization, foregrounds the centrality of medicalization to this book. Medicalization is the process whereby we transform nonmedical parts of life into treatable, curable, illnesses or diseases vis-à-vis medicine and medical frameworks.[29] When we invoke medicalization, we are suggesting that overzealousness to problematize normal parts of the human experience and conceptualize them as medical problems is a mistake. As bioethicist Erik Parens describes this problem, "Living well requires that we learn to let some sorts of problems be. It requires that we learn to affirm, rather than try to erase, variations in our moods, behaviors, and appearances."[30] Yet leaving problems be is, seemingly, antithetical to responsible neoliberal citizenship, wherein we are encouraged to assert control over our health, our minds, and use whatever means are accessible to us to do so. The medicalization of mental states is troubling, therefore, for reasons beyond potentially inflating the numbers of persons with mental disorders (which is then used, in turn, to justify the technologization of mental health): it necessitates that we enact and engage in new regimes and practices to "fix" ourselves, regardless of whether anything is even "wrong" with us to begin with. As psychiatrist Allen Frances suggests, we are witnessing an "expanding concept of mental disorder," leading to a series of

> unfortunate unintended consequences. Only about 5% of the general population has a severe mental disorder; the additional 15–20% have milder and/or more temporary conditions that are placebo responsive and often difficult to distinguish from the expectable problems of everyday life. Yet an amazing 20% of the US population now takes a psychotropic drug and psychotropic drugs are star revenue producers—in the US alone $18 billion/year for anti-psychotics, $12 billion for antidepressants, and $8 billion for ADHD drugs. And 80% of psychotropic drugs are prescribed by primary care physicians with little training and insufficient time to make an accurate diagnosis. There are now more overdoses and deaths from prescribed drugs than from street drugs.[31]

The technologization of mental health is as much about possible futures as it is about the here and now. Responsible citizenship practices, enacted in the present, might be performed not because we are currently experiencing mental distress, but because they are envisioned as preventative measures, undertaken now to avoid psychiatric distress some day in the future. This anticipatory regime evokes Levina and Quinn's description of pre-patients, persons who are not (currently) showing symptoms of illness or disorder but who, someday, might.[32] Yet as disability scholars have long told us, we are all already "at risk" of becoming disabled or ill in the future.[33] Participation in technologized mental health practices, even those that claim to be preventative, does not guarantee able-bodiedness or psychiatric health indefinitely. Nonetheless the assumption is that partaking in these regimes will render us healthier—or at the very least, no sicker—than we already are. Our compliance with this series of assumptions, demonstrated by our utilization of mental health technologies, illustrates that we are willing to see ourselves not only as responsible for our own mental health, but also accepting of responsibility for how our actions affect global economic health and futures.

Neuroplasticity and Medicalization

These anticipatory regimes related to mental health practices did not appear out of nowhere, and their emergence owes much to the popularization of neuroplasticity discourses in medicine and popular culture. Until about 1970 the widespread belief among medical professionals was that the human brain was unalterable by the end of early childhood. This perspective changed dramatically by the end of the twentieth century, however, at which point "the brain had come to be envisaged as mutable across the whole lifespan, open to environmental influences, damaged by insults, and nourished and even reshaped by stimulation—in a word *plastic*."[34]

The significance of this shift in medical and popular conceptualizations of the brain has been profound, as neuroplasticity has come to be deployed as a means of (supposed) empowerment. If the brain is indeed plastic, then by extension we can shape and mold it as necessary. Neuroplasticity therefore facilitates our acceptance of personal responsibility for our brains, our mental health, cognitive functioning, and, by extension, our global economic future. To that effect Rose and Abi-Rached note that if "*we* could rewire our brains . . . The plastic brain becomes a site of choice, prudence, and responsibility *for each individual*."[35] Thanks to neuroplasticity, no longer are our minds beyond our own grasp and management, requiring the help of medical or mental health professionals. Even members of the general, non-expert population, can change our brains—and our lives—by partaking in an array of self-directed practices, involving tools that are marketed and sold on direct-to-consumer markets.

Widespread acceptance of neuroplasticity as fact led to the rise of what have come to be known as "brain training" programs, wherein various activities are believed to improve cognitive functioning. Brain training's underlying premise is that the mind can be strengthened through exercise, much like the rest of the body.[36]

Brain training itself is not new, however, despite how neatly it complements recent neuroplasticity discourses. During the early twentieth century, for instance, a brain training technique known as Pelmanism became wildly popular around the globe.[37] Nonetheless, today there now exists a thoroughly saturated market of brain training tools and technologies that include websites, smartphone applications, and video games. While these are often claimed to result in positive benefits for users, those assertions are based on very little peer-reviewed scholarship.[38] Additionally, whether brain training is useful in the treatment or prevention of mental disorders remains questionable, as research exploring that possibility yields mixed results.[39] What the popularization of brain training has facilitated, however, are increasingly unclear demarcations between what constitutes "normal" and/or "deficient" brain functioning and, relatedly, satisfactory and/or subpar cognitive and mental health. If we believe that responsible neoliberal citizenship practices involve perpetual "work" on our (plastic) brains, then we have also accepted that our brains, in their natural (untrained) states are underoptimized. An untrained brain therefore presents a problem, but one we are told we can fix ourselves. Neuroplasticity thereby perpetuates medicalization of the brain, and this medicalization lends itself to psychiatrization.

Through the lens of neoliberal responsibilization, to choose not to exert control over one's mental health by refusing to partake in technologized regimes and practices to train and "improve" the brain, indicates refusal to be a responsible neoliberal citizen. Others have previously written about the ways in which responsibilization is an integral part of enacting "good" neoliberal citizenship.[40] This book contributes to those conversations by demonstrating the centrality of neoliberalism to the popularization of mental health technologies, particularly through its emphasis upon the individuation of responsibility.

Culture and Mental Health

Mental health's technologization is a microcosm of digital health more broadly, a domain that encompasses "a wide range of technologies related to health and medicine. . . . There are many technologies that come under the rubric of digital health, from those directed at individuals to those used at the population level."[41] In light of digital health's expansion across all domains, one may wonder, why is mental health's technologization worthy of a book unto itself? In addition to discourses and practices resulting from neuroplasticity's intersections with neoliberal practices and beliefs, culture plays a unique role in assessment of what constitutes mental "health" and "illness" that do not hold true for other diseases and disorders.

For one thing, mental health professionals[42] face challenges that are distinct from other medical professions. "Unlike pediatrics or geriatrics, psychiatry does not define itself by reference to a specific demographic population," psychiatrist Warren Kinghorn writes, adding:

> Unlike general surgery or anesthesiology or radiology, it does not define itself exclusively with reference to specific technologies or interventional practices. . . . Unlike certain medical specialties such as nephrology or cardiology, psychiatry cannot lay exclusive claim to a particular body part or organ system. . . . Nor can psychiatry define itself according to a particular institutional structure of practice, since psychiatrists have long shed their historic identification with inpatient institutions and now work within a broad and diverse array of practice settings.[43]

Yet another area of contention exists in regard to how mental disorders might best be understood. While some argue that a biomedical model is best suited to understanding (and by extension, treating) mental illnesses,[44] others emphasize the need to situate diagnoses within specific cultural contexts. Instead these persons might advocate for the practice of "cultural psychology," an approach seeking to reverse the belief that psychology is acultural.[45] As clinical psychologist Pamela Hays notes, the status quo has long been that culture is "a separate category of human experience that only complicates one's understanding of people."[46] In turn, Hays writes:

> [the] marginalization of cultural considerations—particularly those related to minority groups—pervades the field of psychology. Mainstream psychological research still ignores the centrality of culture and separates studies that include cultural minorities (or that simply address cultural influences) into the separate domain of cross-cultural or multicultural psychology. . . . Concomitantly, the most influential psychotherapies (i.e., psychodynamic, behavioral, cognitive-behavioral, humanistic, existential, and family systems) were developed with little and/or highly biased consideration of people seen as being different from the majority of psychologists (whether by ethnicity, nationality, religion, age, sexual orientation, disability, or gender).[47]

To that effect, consider the findings of a comparative study demonstrating the centrality of culture in understanding mental disorders. In this research, participants from India and Ghana, all of whom were diagnosed with schizophrenia, described hearing "voices" as positive experiences, attributing them to their family, friends, or spirits. Yet American participants, also diagnosed with schizophrenia, never described hearing voices positively. Instead they described those voices "as bombardment and as symptoms of a brain disease caused by genes or trauma."[48]

We can also point to the social function of diagnoses of mental disorder as necessitating consideration of cultural context, particularly the ways in which they have been utilized to perpetuate oppression and marginalization, historically and today.[49] Those working in the fields of neurodiversity and mad studies, for example, argue that *disorder, illness,* and related terms pathologize neurological and cognitive differences while also contributing to ableism.[50] Their efforts are often aligned with disability activism, highlighting the harms caused by diagnostic labels and psychiatric treatment protocols in the process of "othering" those persons to whom they are applied.[51] As McWade, Milton, and Beresford describe, "those politically aligned with the psychiatric survivor movement tend to reject medical concepts of their distress and as such would not consider themselves to be psychologically impaired, whereas the social model of disability tends to be read as maintaining impairment to be a biological fact."[52]

Yet psychiatrization, and the oppression which psychiatrization can facilitate, far predates disability and neurodiversity activists' efforts. In slaveholding America, for example, diagnoses of "drapetomania" were used to explain why enslaved persons attempted to escape, as drapetomania was "a disorder of slaves who have a tendency to run away from their owner due to an inborn propensity for wanderlust."[53] Even earlier, Plato hypothesized that women's "wandering wombs" caused discontentment, an assertion that has subsequently lent itself to centuries of gendered pathologizations on the basis of womanhood.[54] What we attempt to explain and understand through medical frameworks is based upon social values, norms, and customs, none of which are infallible or static.[55] To that effect American psychologist Gary Greenberg has noted that, although "drapetomania was never considered for the *Diagnostic and Statistical Manual of Mental Disorders* . . . that may be only because there was no such book in 1850."[56]

Culture's role in determining what constitutes mental disorder and illness is indeed profound. In turn culture, particularly cultural norms and practices, paved the way for technologized regimes of self-care to gain popularity in the domain of mental health. As such, this book foregrounds mental health technologies as simultaneously cultural objects that embody intersecting beliefs about responsibilization and neuroplasticity, as well as tool sets that actively facilitate practices related to medicalization and psychiatrization.

Interdisciplinary Interventions and Research Methodologies

This book provides an interdisciplinary intervention, drawing together a number of traditions and paradigms in pursuit of understanding the relationship between technology, neoliberalism, labor, mental health, and culture. Alongside scholarship from disability studies, bioethics, the medical humanities, and media studies, this book also utilizes theories and insights generated by those working in the fields of science and technology studies

(STS), digital health studies, critical data studies, and critical code and software design, which often highlight the negative, widespread effects of technologies upon social and cultural systems. Although there are no definitive parameters for what constitute these fields, as their objects of inquiry and methods transcend disciplinary boundaries, this work brings together sociologists, anthropologists, communication and media studies scholars, legal theorists, and more in exploration and examinations of the ways in which technologies shape beliefs, ideologies, and behavior.

Some existing scholarship in this vein examines the effects of big data practices,[57] the ways in which algorithms construct our beliefs about world,[58] the effects of surveillance technologies,[59] digital health practices and their relationships to and with neoliberalism,[60] artificial intelligence's effects,[61] and the ways in which media platforms endeavor new labor practices.[62] Quite often this work foregrounds the ways in which technologies perpetuate marginalization and oppression with an eye to gender, race, socioeconomic status, and other aspects of identity. Ruha Benjamin, for example, describes the pervasiveness of discriminatory technologies as "the New Jim Code," highlighting the interconnectedness of historical, race-based segregation with contemporary technological practices and their effects.[63] Safiya Noble's book *Algorithms of Oppression* details a process referred to as "technological redlining," wherein search engines' algorithms engage in profiling of users by gender and race.[64] Simone Browne has written about the surveillance of black bodies and technology's role in facilitating those practices,[65] and Lisa Nakamura's work on internet "cybertypes" highlights how nonwhite persons are stereotyped in digital spaces.[66] Although claims of proprietary knowledge are often deployed to prevent scholars and activists from analyzing technologies, algorithms, and big data sets directly, we instead look to their social, cultural, and otherwise visible effects once they are implemented or released. That is the mode of analysis undertaken throughout this book.

The research presented herein was conducted over a period of roughly five years and utilized a variety of methods. My methodological choices were largely informed by the disciplines of communication studies and anthropology and, more particularly, by approaches that might best be described as feminist research practices. Although what it means to employ a "feminist methodology" has no definitive answer,[67] there is general consensus that such an approach necessitates consideration of matters of voice, power, and reflexivity by researchers.[68] These were particularly salient matters to me as I conducted interviews.[69] Rather than understand my positionality as a researcher as somehow "above" that of any participant, for example, I framed the interviews used in this book as collaborative experiences. I was honest with myself—and interviewees—about my knowledge (or lack thereof), and in turn the interview itself became an opportunity for me to learn from and alongside participants. Sometimes participants wanted to learn about this research and my findings, which I willingly shared with them. Other times, when the opportunity was offered, they wanted to examine their own interviews after transcriptions were complete in order to provide clarifications or further information. In essence, interviews were not unidirectional: they included opportunities for feedback and sustained engagement as a means to facilitate collaborative learning.

The fieldwork I conducted at industry and academic conferences devoted to matters of technology and health, also presented in this book, utilized ethnographic methods. At other times information presented herein was generated from autoethnographic methods as I—like many other feminist researchers—believe that personal knowledge, despite being situated, contains valuable information about culture. Following this tradition, the experiences of the researcher become data used for analytic purposes.[70] It is not unusual for feminist ethnographers to find themselves effectively "written into" their scholarship, blurring the lines between themselves as ethnographers and also subjects of their own critical inquiry.[71] In some chapters, therefore, this book includes descriptions of my own experiences while attending conferences and events, and at other times I share my perceptions and experiences using various mental health technologies.

While there has been a significant amount written about internet ethnographies as a research method,[72] much less has been produced related to autoethnographic research in online spaces.

This is an approach that I undertook, which, though new, represents an exciting mode of analysis wherein the digital self, and its encounters and experiences, are understood to possess unique value in relation to knowledge production.[73] Yet unlike research that is conducted face-to-face, internet-based ethnographies are complicated by a number of matters unique to their online context. These include unclear demarcations between what constitute public and private spaces, who (if anyone) owns or controls data that is publicly accessible, whether we should ever quote data that might be traced back to its author, the difficulty in obtaining informed consent in online contexts, and more.[74] Unsurprisingly, therefore, there are ongoing discussions as to what practices constitute ethical research utilizing such data.[75] In light of those debates, in this book I write only about my own experiences in online spaces. Although that information does, at times, include information about my interactions with others, no potentially identifying information about those with whom I interacted is ever included. This approach, while ethical, omits potential avenues for research that might have shed light upon the experiences of others who utilize mental health technologies. For example, this book does not include publicly accessible ratings and evaluations of mental health technologies that are published on platforms like Reddit, the Google Play and iTunes stores, or any other internet message boards or communities. Nonetheless, I believe it is better to avoid utilizing potentially identifying information produced by others if they have not explicitly consented to their data being used for research purposes.

In addition to interviews and ethnographic methods, this book also provides textual analyses of mental health technologies and platforms. Textual analysis allows the researcher to "discern latent meaning, but also implicit patterns, assumptions and omissions of a text. Text is understood in its broader, poststructural, sense as any cultural practice or object that can be 'read.'"[76] While criticisms of textual analysis suggest that it is not comprehensive in scope because it does not include the related elements of production and consumption,[77] its utility renders it an oft-used method nonetheless. As Phillipov points out,

> insistence that empirical research methods access real dimensions of experience that textual approaches can only abstractly theorize ignores the inevitable partiality of all academic studies. . . . Because they find creative ways to articulate experiences that would otherwise be inaccessible to empirical research methods, the use of text-based approaches can improve, rather than weaken, our understanding of popular media and culture.[78]

Book Organization

This book argues that mental health's technologization reflects new and troubling expansions of neoliberalism. It is in this context that the self, understood as the mind, is believed to be not only malleable but also a site apt for perpetual self-improvement. The mind and its relative healthiness (or unhealthiness) are also no longer matters of private concern. Instead the mind's interconnectedness with economic systems and global futures renders it part of a complex web of beliefs and practices that both reflect and perpetuate the individuation of responsibility through new technologies.

It is true that mental health technologies have led to changes and shifts across culture and medicine, changes that are discussed in detail throughout this book. Those changes, however, do not represent a revolution in the overall accessibility and usability of mental healthcare services. Instead they exist in relation to practices and beliefs about the intersections of technology and medicine, including how we understand mental health and illness, what we believe we should do about experiences with mental distress, and whose mental health matters. The findings presented in this research demonstrate that, to our detriment, one of the consequences of mental health's technologization is the perpetuation and exacerbation of mental health disparities due to gender, race, socioeconomic status, and other aspects of identity. In the end, these consequences render the idealized (and likely impossible) state of complete and utter mental health out of reach for those who are poor, people of color, and otherwise excluded from the hegemonic technological imaginary through no fault of their own.

In service of these overarching arguments, each chapter of this book critically examines a different mental health technology, demonstrating inconsistencies between what its proponents claim it can do with what its concrete effects are for those who use, interact with, or are otherwise affected by it. Chapter 1 presents an analysis of smartphone applications that are available from the iTunes and Google Play stores and that claim to improve user mental health. The creators, designers, and consultants to many of the most popular of these applications imagine themselves as revolutionizing what it means to access and receive mental healthcare. Rather than work within the traditional medical model and system, they suggest, we are all empowered by the ability to download these tool sets and use them without the oversight or guidance of mental health professionals. We each become, in essence, a professional in managing our own mental health. Yet the Food and Drug Administration has allowed this industry to exist entirely without regulation, a decision that raises a multitude of concerns regarding data privacy protections and medical efficacy. What's more, textual analyses of applications themselves reveal their systematic erasure of nonwhite bodies from shared imaginings about whose mental health matters.

Chapter 2 introduces the concept of psychosurveillance, an ethos that necessitates new regimes of surveillance-based practices, wherein nonexpert members of the public are encouraged to engage in the monitoring of others' mental states in online contexts. Psychosurveillance is an uncompensated form of labor, I argue, one that is inherently exploitative and potentially psychologically dangerous for those who provide it. The chapter begins by explicating the history of psychosurveillance before providing a discussion of Facebook's suicide-prevention algorithm, describing the company's public-facing statements about mental distress and self-harm, and including a comparative analysis of that public information with leaked company documents. I then analyze two internet-based platforms, 7 Cups of Tea and Crisis Text Line, and demonstrate their utilization of communitarian appeals to mask the inherently exploitative nature of psychosurveillance practices.

Chapter 3 examines three prominent therapeutic chatbots made possible by advances in artificial intelligence: Woebot, Wysa, and Joy. Their presumed legitimacy as mental health interventions is predicated upon the assumption that algorithms, artificial intelligence, and machine learning systems are capable of providing effective health interventions for all users equally. This chapter demonstrates, however, that this belief is not only false, but also damaging. Not only are these chatbots discriminatory in design, even if unintentionally discriminatory, they also reify a technological imaginary wherein the only bodies invited to participate in practices intended to improve and promote mental health are white, female, and young.

Chapter 4 analyzes telemental healthcare, a more particularized domain of telemedicine, in which mental healthcare services are provided by qualified professionals and delivered via communications technologies. By analyzing a combination of industry fieldwork and interviews, I argue that telemental healthcare cannot eliminate preexisting structural barriers to making equitable mental healthcare possible. Instead what telemental healthcare services provide are improvements in the quality of care received by persons who *already* are mental healthcare service recipients. Additionally, for those working as telemental healthcare professionals, their work's technologization renders them participants in the gig economy. Drawn to this field by appeals of flexibility and entrepreneurialism, telemental healthcare providers often find their labor and expertise devalued and denigrated, even by their peers.

This book's final chapter builds upon and synthesizes previous arguments and claims so as to provide cohesive, concluding remarks about not only neoliberalism's transformation of beliefs about the relationship between technology and mental health but also to reiterate that technological interventions are incapable of solving the mental healthcare crisis. I also present a series of predictions about the likely consequences of mental health's technologization, including the fruition of a future wherein mental health technologies become utilized as mechanisms of population management, oppression, and control.

The book concludes with what I have titled a "COVID Coda,"[79] wherein I discuss how the global COVID-19 pandemic made many of the issues related to mental health, technology, and the continued marginalization of persons in need of mental health-care services, all previously addressed in this book, even more pressing. COVID-19 made it abundantly clear that we need no longer only imagine a possible future wherein technological access is a determinant of life and death. We now inhabit a world wherein invisible, uncurable illnesses could potentially kill us, and therefore technologies that allow us to live "safely" are integral to responsible citizenship practices as well as our survival. Yet for those unable to partake in these practices, due to the digital divide and all that it entails, enacting "good" neoliberal citizenship remains an impossibility. Matters of technological accessibility and usability are now, more than ever, determinants of who is invited to partake in citizenship practices. Those without the requisite tools become largely invisible, excluded from our social and cultural imaginaries. By being cast as "noncitizens," they are also dehumanized.

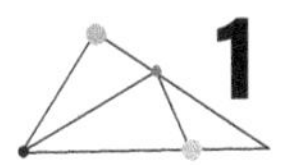

1

Mental Wellness by Smartphone App

In 2009 Apple debuted its first commercial for smartphone applications (described as "apps") in the following televised advertisement:

> What's great about the iPhone is that if you want to check snow conditions on the mountain, there's an app for that. If you want to check how many calories are in your lunch, there's an app for that. And if you want to check where exactly you parked the car, there's even an app for that. Yep. There's an app for just about anything. Only on the iPhone.[1]

Although the applications described in the commercial might seem dated in comparison to many that are now available, it nonetheless contains an ongoing truism: apps are often used with the intent to improve ourselves, particularly in matters of health.

In 2009 the abilities of applications to do so, however, were limited by their technological capacities. As the commercial states, "check[ing] how many calories are in your lunch" by inputting information into an app was, at the time, novel and exciting. Today advances in widely available technologies have made it possible to simply photograph food in order for an app to determine its caloric information.[2] What's more, interest in applications to facilitate self-improvement has expanded far beyond calorie counting. Now apps can aid us in all sorts of health-related domains, including tracking ovulation cycles, menstruation, and fertility;[3] monitoring water intake and urine quality;[4] informing us whether we eat too quickly,[5] have repellant body odor,[6] or are sleeping poorly;[7] or, as is the subject of this chapter, how we can better track, manage, and improve our mental health.

Today there are roughly 22,750 applications that claim to improve user mental health and are available for free (or at low cost) through the iTunes and Google Play stores.[8] Some of their creators assert that their efficacy results from utilizing therapeutic techniques such as cognitive behavioral therapy (CBT), a strategy that emphasizes teaching individuals to learn to recognize and modify their own unhealthy thinking patterns.[9] There are also mental health applications that have been evaluated in research trials, in hopes of demonstrating beyond a doubt that they provide effective mental health outcomes for users.[10] Other applications provide guided meditations, spaces for daily journaling, thought exercises, and contemplation prompts, bolstered by preexisting research about the benefits of meditation and mindfulness practices.[11]

Yet this immense variability among mental health applications actually reflects a significant problem. In the United States the Food and Drug Administration (FDA) does not regulate health applications, claiming that they should be understood solely as mobile applications and not mobile *medical* applications. The FDA regulates only the latter category and insists that any app distributed through the iTunes or Google Play stores does not constitute a medical device, regardless of its claims of efficacy.[12] This determination by the FDA comes at a cost. Without oversight or regulation, smartphone applications that are designed, marketed, and sold directly to consumers for the purposes of managing or improving their health are not required to undergo any sort of vetting process. If any evaluations are made of these tools, they are made by consumers themselves.

Despite the lack of FDA oversight, the American Psychiatric Association (APA) does not discourage the use of mental health applications, nor is its position that mental health professionals should discourage their utilization. Instead the APA suggests a series of evaluative questions for mental healthcare providers to use in determining, again on an individual basis, whether an application might benefit a patient. Suggested dimensions for consideration include background about the app and whether its claims about outcomes are realistic, consideration of data privacy concerns, assessing ease of usability, and whether practitioners can access data that patients share with—or is autonomously collected by—the app.[13]

An entirely different approach was undertaken in the United Kingdom, where the National Health Service (NHS) has attempted to regulate health applications by creating a Health Apps Library. This initiative intends to evaluate and rate applications claiming to improve user health, and has even included a separate division for mental health applications.[14] The program was temporarily shuttered in 2015 when it was discovered that even many of its "approved" applications did not protect the data, privacy, and identities of persons who had downloaded and used them.[15] The Health Apps Library was rebooted in 2017, however, with renewed dedication to vetting applications prior to granting a seal of approval.[16] While regulation and monitoring of consumer-facing health applications, and more particularly mental health applications, is clearly possible, the FDA's hands-off approach is reflective of a neoliberal ethos: we are all responsible not only to manage our health vis-à-vis technologies but also for ascertaining which technologies are even useful to begin with.

This book's introduction explicated the relationship between neoliberalism, health technologies, neuroplasticity, and medicalization. In this chapter I build upon that framework in the context of smartphone applications, highlighting their unique role in expanding beliefs about responsibilization while also endeavoring new regimes of practices related to (mental) self-care practices. Whereas existing scholarship on mental health applications explores their ability to provide medically beneficial outcomes to users[17] this chapter details the ways in which proponents of mental health applications, including their designers, company founders, and consultants, conceptualize and articulate their legitimacy. Prior to that, however, I share my experiences at two conferences for persons working at the intersections of health and technology: WinterTech, and Technology, the Mind and Society.

The WinterTech and Technology, the Mind and Society Conferences

On January 11, 2017, I attended the third annual WinterTech conference. It was a one-day event hosted by the digital health company Health 2.0, which "promotes, showcases and catalyzes new technologies in health care . . . bring[ing] together the best minds, resources and technology for compelling panels, discussions and product demonstrations, and more."[18] The organization's cofounders Indu Sabaiya and Matthew Holt, who possess backgrounds in medicine and healthcare technologies,[19] facilitated the event during San Francisco's noted J. P. Morgan Healthcare Conference, an annual gathering largely regarded as the healthcare industry's premier investment symposium.[20]

WinterTech was held at the Julia Morgan Ballroom, an elegant venue in San Francisco's Merchants Exchange building. Designed in the Beaux-Arts style, intricate carvings and details adorned the space's walls, ceilings, and fireplaces; oversized windows provided sweeping views of the city; and its seventeen-foot-high ceilings were ornamented with ornate chandeliers.[21] Although I have been to many professional conferences in my life, I had never been to any quite so glamorous. It was clear from the money spent on the conference space alone that the business of digital health was booming. Beginning with a 7 a.m. invite-only breakfast for technologists and potential financial investors, the rest of the day's events featured a variety of panels, technology demonstrations, and fireside chats (interviews with notable industry figures) to discuss how the field of digital health would likely grow and evolve during the upcoming year.

WinterTech was entirely technocentric, premised upon the belief that positive changes in health systems result from empowering consumers, and that in order to empower them, we must place health technologies directly in their hands. This orientation toward technology's role in the healthcare ecosystem diverges from the traditional model, wherein practitioners and clinicians must first accept technologies themselves before integrating them into their workflows and interactions with patients. Yet WinterTech attendees and speakers explicitly espoused the sentiment that health technologies, in order to be successful, should disrupt (even dismantle) this status quo. As a number of the conference's invited speakers mentioned, however, this paradigm shift creates tension between technologists and healthcare industry professionals, as the latter are unlikely to be open to technologies that change the traditional power relationships between patients and providers. As a result, a number of WinterTech speakers predicted that, despite the utility and efficacy of many technologies that were discussed that day, governing bodies and organizations in medicine would be uninterested in promoting their adoption. It was therefore the responsibility of technologists and consumers to advocate for change.

While there was much discourse about revolutionizing health practices and healthcare systems at WinterTech, I was troubled by an absence of discussion about how, exactly, any new, exciting, or revolutionary technology might actually be placed into consumers' hands. I do not believe that there was a single session dedicated to discussion or exploration of matters related to distribution, access, and equity. Instead, while the conference emphasized disruption of the medical industry status quo, it did so without consideration of how we might similarly "disrupt" the digital divide, or the gap between those able to access technologies and those who cannot.[22] Even the conference's keynote, which addressed affordable and accessible healthcare, and was provided by president and CEO of Blue Shield of California Paul Markovich, never mentioned the digital divide or obstacles related to the accessibility of technologies. During the Q&A portion of Markovich's talk, I therefore felt compelled to ask how, if at all, he imagined the digital divide might affect access to healthcare technologies if the presumption was that technologies themselves democratize access to healthcare services. Markovich's response seemed to be a deflection. "Yes, it's an issue," he stated, but added that technology "creates an incentive for health plans to bridge that gap." He then moved on. At no point that day was there further discussion of how we might not only create technologies but also "bridge that gap" between those who can access them and those who cannot.

Markovich was wrong. The mere existence of a technology does not create an incentive for an entity to strive for equitable distribution of that technology. Consider that in the introduction to this book I described a number of insurance companies' "incentives" for members to adopt and use self-tracking technologies, incentives that included discounts on insurance plans. Yet none of those technologies were provided to plan enrollees, or enrollees' dependents, for free. Some of those plans offered technologies at discounted rates, but they were not free, despite the fact that insurance companies benefit when their members use them. Once again, we see risk and responsibilization offset onto the shoulders of individual, private citizens, even when the economic benefits are to corporations and not us. Not only are we encouraged to utilize technologies as part of responsible citizenship practices, we are also told that it is our responsibility to acquire the requisite technologies in the first place. Those who cannot afford to purchase or otherwise access them, despite their desire to do so, are thereby precluded from participating in these regimes of neoliberal responsibilization.

My hope for WinterTech had been that presentations or discussions might include some mention of mental health technologies, and I admit that I was surprised by the lack of discourse about them. Mental illness came up only once, and very briefly, during a fireside chat with Jessica Mega of Verily, a subsidiary of Alphabet that develops health technologies.[23] Mega, while reflecting upon the vast number of self-tracking technologies able to generate smart data for an array of disorders and illnesses, remarked in passing that it is our current inability to generate smart data about mental health and illness that precludes such technologies from events like WinterTech. Though brief, Mega's point was significant, as it emphasized an often unstated paradox about mental health applications that incorporate tracking functions: they assume that there is utility in tracking our mental states, although there is no evidence to suggest that big data can be reliably used to improve and manage our mental health.

Before continuing, an explication of terminology is warranted. "Big data" is a phrase used across multiple industries and disciplines to describe the vast amounts of information collected about us by a variety of electronic information systems, including social networks, mobile devices, electronic health records, and more.[24] Sometimes that information is collected autonomously by machine intelligence, whereas at other times it might be input manually. Regardless, big data's utility results from its ability to be used for analysis. When vast amounts of data are organized in such a way that they have predictive value, and by extension are useful in decision-making processes by algorithms or humans, they constitute what is referred to as "smart data."[25]

Yet there are reasons to be concerned about big data, smart data, and their use in any health domain. Legal scholars, for example, point out the likelihood of data privacy violations by any entities that collect and analyze data about us.[26] There remains a very real possibility that information about us will be "collected by data trackers, combined with other data, analyzed, and re-sold as data products by data brokers."[27] Even so, today about one in three people tracks information about their health with either a smartphone application or a wearable device.[28] Privacy concerns related to big data collection and analysis, however, should be considered even more pressing in the context of mental disorders and illnesses, due to their particularly stigmatized nature.

In addition to data privacy, applications for mental health improvement are concerning for yet another reason: there is currently no scientific justification in tracking mental states for the purpose of generating smart data. There are a number of studies underway that seek to correlate biodata (such as heart rate) with mental distress and illness. At the time of writing, however, the efficacy of these initiatives remains unproven. Nevertheless, support for digital phenotyping in the domain of mental health, a process whereby smart data would be used to diagnose and monitor mental health and illness,[29] persists. Researchers have, for example, tested wearable patches intended to correlate stress levels (measured through heart rate, sleep patterns, and so forth) with mental distress and illness,[30] and there are also apps that analyze how persons' interactions and engagements with their phones can be used to evaluate their mental states.[31] Some suggest that we need not even create additional applications and software to generate smart data about our mental states, as our smartphones' passive sensing technologies will soon be able to

> include intervention components such as notifications when an individual is aroused (e.g., through galvanic skin response, heart rate variability, etc.) to engage in stress-management techniques or . . . alerts based on GPS or geographic information

> to avoid high-risk situations. . . . With new voice capture and analysis technologies becoming more commonplace . . . to assess the emotional tone of speech or use text recognition software to assess depressive or other symptomology . . . [and] facial scans to determine emotion from subtle facial cues.[32]

Nonetheless, for the time being the pursuit of smart data about mental health, even as a byproduct of smartphones' processes, is unwarranted. These approaches therefore reflect techno-solutionist beliefs based upon anticipatory logics, not grounded in present realities.

Despite WinterTech's lack of discourse about mental health technologies, I imagined that efforts to create and discuss such interventions must be happening, even if they were happening elsewhere. My search led me to learn of the upcoming inaugural Technology, Mind and Society (TMS) conference, organized by the American Psychological Association and to be held in Washington, D.C., during the spring of 2018. I decided to attend.

The TMS conference was impressive, not just due to its grandiose location at the Marriott Marquis, but also the sheer number of experts in the fields of psychology, robotics, artificial intelligence, and human–computer interaction who were scheduled to provide its keynotes and presentations. Despite being the first-ever TMS meeting, the conference drew roughly four hundred attendees from thirty countries, all with shared interest in technology's ability to shape knowledge and practices related to mental health and illness. TMS was also devotedly multidisciplinary. Though sponsored by the American Psychological Association, presenters and attendees hailed from many fields, including robotics, computer science, cybersecurity, and education, all of whom were drawn together by their shared belief in the capacity of technologies to improve mental health.

The conference's opening reception was held in the Marquis's largest ballroom, where tables were piled high with macarons, cupcakes, risotto, coffee, and tea. Complimentary wine and beer were also available to attendees at bars that were scattered throughout the room. Just after six in the evening Dr. Arthur C. Evans,

CEO of the American Psychological Association, took to the stage. He began by describing how his own interest in the intersections of psychology and technology had started thirty years earlier while in graduate school, and how excited he was by where the field was headed today. At the heart of technology's implementation into the field of psychology, Evans emphasized, is "human behavior. And that's why we at APA are so interested in that topic and are delighted to do this conference. And whether you're talking about the models on which much of this technology is developed . . . or the interaction between technology and people, or the impact that this technology has upon society and people, at the heart of that, often is the issue of psychology. And so, we really hope that tonight is the beginning of our work, as an association, in this area."

The opening night's keynote was provided by Dr. Cynthia Breazeal, who is widely considered one of the most prominent and forward-thinking researchers in social robots and human–robot interactions. The following morning attendees were given another presentation from Microsoft's chief scientific officer Dr. Eric Horvitz, an expert in machine intelligence. Other featured talks were provided by Dr. Justine Cassell, now the inaugural international chair at PRAIRIE (Paris Institute on Interdisciplinary Research in AI), and Dr. Alex Pentland, MIT's Toshiba Professor and, according to *Forbes,* one of the "most powerful data scientists in the world."[33] TMS also included a number of smaller-scale panel presentations, discussions, and sponsored sessions that examined an array of phenomena, including racial biases in first-person-shooter games, wearable devices meant to improve suicide prevention efforts, the effects of smartphone usage upon well-being, humans' emotional relationships with robots, the utility of tactile robots in treating developmental disorders, the therapeutic value of virtual reality, and much, much more.

Yet there were times during the conference that I found showcased technologies and interventions concerning. At one panel presentation, for example, researchers from the University of Pennsylvania shared an algorithm that they described as "prediagnostic," claiming that it could diagnose attention deficit hyperactivity disorder (ADHD) in Twitter users based upon the content of their posts. When the talk concluded, I asked the presenting researcher whether a predictive model for a mental disorder seemed, in his view, at all problematic. My hope was that his response would speak to some of my concerns related to the nature of the algorithm and the team's methods, such as data privacy, the (non-)consent of persons whose data were used for its development, and the possibility of the algorithm being used to diagnose persons without their consent. I was surprised when the presenter seemed to appear uncomfortable, as I had assumed that he and his team would have considered and been prepared for the possibility of such a question from one, if not more, audience members. His response, in essence, was that any data, once shared online, is effectively public property. This rendered his team's collection and analysis justified. Although he added that he did not want this tool to get into what he termed the "wrong hands," he noted that the project's approval by his university's institutional approval board (IRB) meant that their work was ethical.

I did not ask any follow-up questions. Instead I thanked the presenter for his response. Initiating a public debate at a prestigious conference, when I worried that my concerns were not likely shared with others in the room, was not my intent, despite how thoroughly I took issue with the response I was given. First and foremost, approval by an institution's IRB should not be considered a reflection of its ethicality. Many research projects, despite being approved by IRBs, are unethical.[34] Second, debates are ongoing as to what constitutes private versus public data, even in the context of Twitter and other "open" internet forums.[35] This is a particularly pressing consideration in the context of mental disorders, which continue to be highly stigmatized. Yet that this research team's position was that the data they used was unquestioningly "public" left no opportunity to consider my concerns legitimate.

In pursuit of further clarity since my attendance at TMS, I looked into the fate of the ADHD-predicting algorithm. I found that its creators had published an article in the *Journal of Attention Disorders* and was disappointed to find that ethical questions and concerns related to its development and implementation were only raised in a brief paragraph in the article's conclusion:

> The feasibility of social-media-based assessment of ADHD also raises ethical questions. Employers and insurance companies, for example, may be motivated to assess people using their social media. As ADHD may be viewed as a "mental illness" and carry social stigma and may engender discrimination, data protection and ownership frameworks are needed to make sure the data are not used against the users' interest. . . . Few users realize the amount of mental-health-related information that can be gleaned from their digital traces, so transparency about which indicators are derived by whom for what purpose should be part of ethical and policy discourse.[36]

It is possible that others at the TMS conference, if asked questions about mental health technologies, data privacy, and ethics, might have responded differently than those who created this diagnostic algorithm. And, I admit, my question during the presentation and ongoing concerns highlight problems without easy or definitive solutions and answers. Yet as I reflect upon my experiences at WinterTech and TMS in tandem, what stands out most in my memory are the disquieting gaps and absences in discourse about mental health technologies. I am, of course, speaking in generalities about my overall impressions, as I was not able to attend every single session or presentation. However, based upon what I did see and hear at those conferences, I am struck by what was missing from them: concern with matters of equity, accessibility, and data privacy. I am reminded as well of the Facebook company's original motto: "Move fast and break things."[37] The speed at which we are "moving" in the realm of mental health technologies is far greater than the speed at which we are able to comprehend all of the implications and effects those technologies have upon their users and society more broadly. Yet by sidelining those concerns, particularly at prominent industry and academic conferences, we reify the notion that they *deserve* to be sidelined, that they are secondary to our ability to innovate. I am concerned that all of this foreshadows a future wherein critique, questioning, and thoughtful discourse about technologies' effects are ignored, brushed aside, and systematically disregarded.

I hope I am wrong.

Interviews with Applications' Advocates

Despite a lack of conference-sponsored discourse about the ethically suspect dimensions of mental health technologies, I imagined that there might still be others who shared my concerns. I also considered the possibility that those who were more familiar with the ins and outs of mental health technologies, such as smartphone apps, might share information and perspectives that would assuage my worries. I conducted a series of interviews with persons working in the field of mental health applications, not only to discover whether I was alone in my trepidations about those tools, but also to learn how industry members themselves conceptualized and understood their work.

Motivated by Personal Need

Some of those who agreed to participate in interviews possessed backgrounds in mental health; others were technologists, data scientists, and software engineers. Despite those differences, many shared a similar narrative: they had been drawn to the field of mental health applications because of a personal need for mental health interventions that were both discreet and portable. Yet, as no such technologies had been available to them, they set about creating them, first for themselves, and then for a commercial market.

Consider what I was told by Charles, a computer programmer who developed an app for anxiety. He explained that his motivation to create an application was due to "personal experience . . . I developed this app primarily for myself with a little hope that it could be of some help to others as well." Levi, another application creator, offered a parallel explanation:

> The original idea was that I had anxiety myself. I was looking at mobile apps that I could use for my own anxiety. And in doing so, I found that they were either clinical, so they were either developed by clinicians (but those usually didn't have very wide adoption), and then on the other side they had mainstream relaxation apps that did have wide adoption but they weren't using the clinical tool sets. . . . I kind of felt like I had a unique understanding of consumer design and also

> what it was like to go through anxiety. And the idea was sort of, what if we take clinical tools, distill them to their simplest parts, and take some of that consumer edge from the relaxation app, and kind of combine that? Where would we be?

Jordan, also an application founder, shared a similar experience: "I was trying to learn meditation practices, and body scanning techniques, and really learning how to calm my mind down. . . . So as I talked to a colleague about what exactly it was that we were going to be building [in the app], we found out that a lot of the tools that therapists use are very similar to some of things I was trying to teach myself."

The entrepreneurial spirit suggested by these stories reflects the privatization and individuation of responsibility in matters of mental health. App creators and founders knew what they wanted, and what they believed they medically needed, to improve their own mental health. Unable to find those tools, they created them themselves.

All of the interviewees with whom I spoke offered success stories, in the sense that the interventions offered by their respective apps were positively received by users. Yet this evidences a state of affairs wherein interviewees had come to understand their psychological distress as their own responsibility, not only due to its personal nature and origins, but also because it necessitated self-directed solutions. It is vital, therefore, that even as we applaud innovators, we should not decontextualize their technologies from the contexts in which they emerge. In this case, the neoliberal ethos of responsibilization made interviewees, and the rest of us, complicit in perpetuating a falsehood: that we are individually responsible not only for the origins of our mental distress but also for generating solutions to the problems our distress creates.

Legitimizing Mental Health Applications

As discussed previously in this book, the distinctions between what constitute states of mental health and disorder are increasingly unclear, due in part to medicalization and psychiatrization, but also culture's role in defining what states are markedly "ill" and/or "healthy." Regardless, mental health applications are positioned by their proponents as interventions for improving mental health, maintaining mental healthiness, as well as preventing the onset of mental illness. In such a way they are emblematic of neoliberalism's concern with multiple temporalities, including the present and the possible futures. Therefore, regardless of one's relationship to mental distress (that is to say, whether we experience it already or are simply at risk of experiencing it someday), these applications are framed by their advocates as useful for us all.

Levi noted, for example, that many of his application's users are "using our tool set as a stand-alone, [to] sort of self-care, self-manage their life." Some, he added, come to

> realize that they want to seek professional help, so then [the app] sort of serves as a catalyst getting them into therapy. And then there's a lot of people that are just using it alongside their weekly therapist appointment. And so, you know, we're kind of, we're already straddling both worlds where we're a consumer app on one side for people that aren't necessarily in therapy, but we're also a clinical app for people that are in therapy.

That an application functions "as a catalyst [for] getting them into therapy" would seemingly establish its legitimacy as an effective mental health intervention. I applaud any person who recognizes that they are experiencing distress and seeks professional care. Yet Levi's comment also demonstrates that mental health applications serve a medicalizing function, encouraging users to understand themselves as mentally ill or disordered, for two reasons. First, all of those who utilize these apps do so with intentionality. That is to say, their use reflects acceptance of their own subjectivity as in need of some sort of mental health intervention, even if that subjectivity is self-imposed. Secondarily, by utilizing a "treatment" (in this case, an application) that treats all users the same, and that is designed and intended for users who are indeed in need of a mental health intervention, it will likely lead users to believe that they *are* in need of mental health interventions. Although, of course, it is better to seek out mental healthcare services that are unnecessary than to risk going without them, my concerns about the consequences of the medicalization of mental states and psychiatrization of the human condition, discussed in the introduction to this book, persist nonetheless.[38]

Another legitimation strategy discussed by interviewees was their utilization of research trials. These were presented to me as concrete evidence that mental health applications offer measurable, positive outcomes for their users, regardless of whether they experience mental distress or illnesses, or should be understood as subclinical. Mary, a licensed psychologist who works as consultant to a popular application, spoke in depth about the necessity of clinical trials. Prior to her current position she had worked with another mental health app developer but left when they claimed that rigorous, scientific research and testing would never be possible for an app:

> They basically told me that, you know, they would never be willing to do good science because it's not realistic to have control groups. . . . But now the company I'm with really is serious about science. So when they convinced me they were serious about science, then we started really talking. So I was there from the very beginning, and the goal was to come up with the product that conveyed only rigorously, scientifically tested techniques to the general public.

Others with whom I spoke also emphasized the necessity of clinical research. Yet because they themselves were not mental health professionals or researchers, they relied upon consultants to advise them of best practices. Levi shared, for example, that "when we started off we needed to work side-by-side with professionals. That would be the responsible way to go. . . . And, you know, they're there to make sure that the content is sound, that the tools are sound, and that we're following all of the best practices in the field."

Jordan similarly shared that, from the beginning, he has strived to create a product that is respected by mental health professionals. This, he explained, is "one of the reasons that we've aligned ourselves with clinical practices as much as we can, so that when a professional picks us, they understand exactly what the tool set is and how they can use it." In addition to creating a technology respected by clinicians, he hopes that his application will increasingly become one that practitioners want to incorporate into their patients' treatment plans:

> The next step that we're undergoing is building tools for the mental health professionals, whether they are the counselors, psychologists, psychiatrists, social workers. We take a little bit of a different approach than some of our competitors in that we absolutely do not want to compete against professional therapy, and rather would create a set of tools that they can use to work with their patients in order to really improve the continuum of care, and make sure that they have the right data to inform how they're working with their patient. There are a lot of companies out there that are trying to disrupt the way the mental health industry works, and we don't think that's actually a necessity.

Another legitimation strategy utilized by interviewees was the assertion that there are similarities between mental health apps and other self-tracking technologies. This is despite, as discussed earlier in this chapter, a lack of evidence that the creation of smart data for matters of mental illness is possible. Nonetheless, Levi's comments seemed to suggest this as true:

> When we started off there was a lot of skepticism about, "could you have an app for mental health?" or "could technology really, really make a difference in terms of peoples' mental health?" And I think that even within the past two years a lot more people are understanding that yes, this is a thing, this is true. . . . The same way that people use FitBit and sensors and different things to take care of their physical health, I think that we're going to see the same thing with mental health, where people would rather use an app to work on that and then maybe go into therapy as needed, as opposed to the way it is today.

To the same effect, Jordan also noted that because our smartphones are with us most—if not all—of the time, he had "wanted to create a tool set that was able to track people in the moment . . . it's actually called Ecological Momentary Assessment. So that opportunity to get accurate data from an individual really can help drive the healthcare outcomes in the long run." Again, despite the lack of evidence to show that digital phenotyping is possible in the domain of mental health, this anticipatory perspective reflects the dual orientations of mental health applications: they are to be used in the present, and will become even more useful in the future (should psychiatric smart data ever become a reality).

The Neoliberalization of Application Users

Because they are available through the iTunes and Google Play stores, mental health applications are marketed and sold directly to consumers. As a result, it should come as no surprise that information about application popularity and user retention rates was often referenced by interviewees to demonstrate that their applications are indeed successful. Don, a software engineer, stated that success of the app he built is measured by "the number of users who continue to use the app based on improvement . . . There's millions of users. . . . We can just anonymously see at a very high level that people are improving over time." Levi described his application as being much like any other consumer product:

> Consumer businesses still measure success based on how many sign-ups are you getting, are you retaining your users, how much money are you making from those users. But we tend to think about it—we have a simple metric—and we just think about, "Are we helping people?" And so from the consumer perspective, we know we are helping you based on your mood ratings (so we can tell if people are improving over time). . . . And then we also anecdotally know. We get a lot of praise and love letters about the app itself and how it's helping. So we just try to think about is this going to help somebody manage their stress? Manage their anxiety?

> And if we keep focusing on that, everything else tends to fall into place.

Jordan pointed out that he looks at

> daily user retention. How many people are continuing to use the products on an ongoing basis. It's not necessarily an accurate portrayal because in the healthcare space, if they're really helping people get better, they shouldn't need to use your tools quite as much. So, you know, fundamentally the core metric has to be the value that you provide to the end user, individual. And making sure that you're really helping them improve.

A contradiction evident in this comment is particularly noteworthy. If a technology is causing improvements in a user's health, then seemingly they would need to use and rely upon that technology less. Yet while the data Jordan accesses about his application's users indicates that they are experiencing improvements in their mental health, they continue to use the application consistently. This raises a troubling question: if these tools are improving user mental health, then why don't usage rates drop off once improvements are experienced?

The reason is likely attributable to the cultural function of mental health applications rather than their medical efficacy. These apps' users are committed to using them. They cannot simply "stop" doing so for two reasons. As previously mentioned, they have already accepted their own subjectivity as a person in need of a mental health intervention. By extension, engaging in technologized self-care practices necessitates ongoing investment in their use. Using these tools becomes a regular part of one's neoliberal citizenship practices. We cannot stop being good citizens, and so we cannot stop using the applications that *make us* good citizens.

Good citizenship practices, however, involve more than the individuation of responsibility. To that effect, Mary shared information suggesting the likelihood of a future wherein mental health applications will no longer be marketed and sold directly to consumers, who can presumably choose whether or not to use them, but rather will be integrated into new regimes and practices mandated by employers and insurance companies:

> I think in the beginning we saw ourselves as a consumer-facing platform, so something that consumers would find and subscribe to. . . . We do have a decent number of subscribers but not really enough to sustain the platform, so we've been looking to other ventures, and where I really think that we are going to land is as something that employers and health insurance companies purchase to be given to the people that they're responsible for. So, we've been having conversations with and striking up contracts with health insurance companies, particularly to target particular disorders that are a problem for them. One thing is health insurance companies, they want to reduce their cost usually by reducing distress in particularly health-compromised populations. I think some health insurance companies are also looking at us as an app to give to everybody to reduce costs. . . . Then we also have companies wanting to improve employee well-being because there's all this research to suggest that happy employees do better jobs. Basically, they do better at work. So now it's becoming more of a business-facing platform, and then the business is the one that disseminates it to individuals. We're doing a lot of that now, but the data are not in yet because it's just gotten started. So, we'll see how that plays out.

The evolution of Mary's application, from self-directed technology to (soon-to-be) mandated tool set, was driven by her company's financial needs and goals. Now the impetus to utilize the application is no longer related to individual choice, although "choice" itself is somewhat of misnomer since responsible citizenship would encourage the use of these apps even without directives. However, once the utilization of these applications does become explicitly directed, whatever boundaries once existed between mental health, distress, and disorder will no longer matter. Instead, we will all undergo technologically facilitated, mandated psychiatrization.

Accessibility, Usability, and the Imagined User

During conversations I made sure to ask interviewees about matters of access, particularly whether they believed that their applications increase the accessibility of mental healthcare services. Jordan responded in the affirmative, citing his application's affordability as a reason that it does increase access, and emphasizing its inclusion of elements that are free of charge to users:

> I think the biggest problem that we see is that, if you look at the market as a whole, there are 60 million adults, maybe less, that suffer from mental illness every year. And only a third of them are actually receiving help. So, there's this huge issue of access to care and actually helping people understand that there are tools out there that are available to them. . . . We want to make sure that we're really providing tools for as many people as we can.

In fact, he told me, "98 percent of our users use the free part" of the app's features, adding that this had been "a conscious decision to try to get tools into the hands of individuals." In Jordan's view, the cost of his application (that is, the fact that it is free) is what makes it accessible.

Mary's conceptualization of accessibility was more comprehensive. Although she, like Jordan, mentioned the (low) price of her application, she also emphasized the multidimensional nature of the construct of "access." In comments reflecting upon digital healthcare services more generally, she noted that compared to in-person services, they require

> fewer, less costs, to get there. . . . If I want to see a specialist for anything, I basically have to go to the closest city, so I have to drive. So that assumes I have a car. It assumes I can afford the gas to drive each way. It assumes I can take basically half a day off of work to drive each way. And then the doctor might be terrible, right? . . . If, you know, my internet doctor sucks, I just call another one . . . then five minutes later I'm talking to another one. So [digital healthcare] shortens that gap, which I think is so important. . . . There are all these

> barriers to care and how hard it is. . . . Assuming you are even wanting to seek care, right? Assuming you are overcoming the stigma associated with seeking treatments for something, which many people are not, then you've got all these other [considerations] . . . You've got to physically get there. You still have to pay the co-pay, which you still have to do with these digital [doctors], they cost about the same actually as far as I can tell. . . . So, you know, the cost isn't lower, but all of the costs—the time cost, the effort cost, the disappointment in having to, you know, do things again . . . These online versions of physical and mental healthcare is really an extraordinary opportunity to make the distance between person and the care much, much shorter.

Another dimension of accessibility discussed by Levi is the portability of mental health applications. He noted that

> the idea was that if our product was going to have relaxation tools, tracking tools, and in order for people to actually use those, it has to be in your pocket available all the time, because that was going to be where you need to access those tools. So for example, if somebody was stressed out and needed to do a deep breathing exercise, it seemed more plausible that they would be able to pull out their phone and access it that way as opposed to pulling up a website on their computer.

Portability is not the same as accessibility, but the pervasiveness of their conflation was also evident in my conversation with Don, a programmer who had been contracted by a nonprofit to create their application. He shared the following: "Everybody has these devices on them . . . recording metrics about what people are doing, and how people are being out in the world. . . . I think it's a very powerful thing that everybody has these very smart devices on them and they can reach to them for support at any time." Although Don never actually described who is included in the "everybody" that he mentioned, I surmise that his statements about "access" referred only to persons who already possess the requisite technologies through which mental health apps can be obtained. Nonetheless his comments illustrate the belief that technologies empower us to care for ourselves more effectively than we would be able to without them.

When I pressed interviewees for information about who uses their mental health applications, it became clear that they are technologies of responsibilization intended primarily for—and used by—young, white women. Jordan shared, for example, that the median age of his app's user is twenty-eight, and that roughly 80 percent of the application's users are female. He did add that he believes that this "demographic is going to shift" in the future, though for now the knowledge of who his power users are helps "tailor the consumer application based on sort of what expectations are within that demographic." When I asked Don during our conversation why the guided meditations his application offered were provided by voices that sounded white and female, his response was that he did not "think that was part of any conscious choice." Levi, asked the same question about his application, offered the following:

> We actually tried out a bunch of different voice actors, male and female. We had some that were very relaxing, but people felt were too robotic. We had others that had a lot of humanity in their voice, but people were more alienated by the different accents. So the woman we ended up with was a combination of a soothing voice that also felt like it had some humanity in it, where people could tell this isn't like Siri[39] talking to me, and also they couldn't pick out where she's from. And that ended up being important when, you know, we're definitely being used across the country and across the world. It can be off-putting if somebody's got, you know, like an East Coast accent, Midwest accent, Southern accent. That's easier for people to pick through when they're not from that part of the country. So those are the three criteria for why we ended up with her.

I do not believe it was merely coincidence that, when these interviews were conducted, the most popular mental health applications on the market exclusively utilized voices that sounded white and female. One could argue that the choice to design apps in such a way was a reflection of a shared cultural imaginary, wherein young, white women were representative of the general population. By extension, the design of these mental health applications would therefore reflect that particular identity and its characteristics. Yet such an argument is demonstrably false. It would mean believing that white, female bodies are envisioned as "neutral" bodies. In the context of the United States (where all of the applications discussed with these interviewees were designed) the hegemonic identity is white, yes, but it is the male body that is considered neutral. Therefore, the other, much more likely, explanation for the discrepancy between the neutral body and the bodies that these tools are designed for is that mental health applications are designed to speak to white, young, and female users because they are the ones expected to engage in neoliberal practices of responsibilization more so than any other population. Considered in conjunction with arguments about the gendered expectations that women, much more so than men, are called upon to provide and engage in affective and emotional labor,[40] it becomes all the more clear that these applications perpetuate both gendered and racialized conceptualizations of who should—and ought to—partake in technologically facilitated mental health practices.

The Effects of Nonregulation

Whereas I have already noted my concerns related to the FDA's nonregulation of mental health applications, interviewees were of an altogether different mindset. Jordan, for instance, suggested that the lack of regulation actually represented "support from the FDA . . . It was a conscious decision on their part to help companies like ours. . . . And I think we're going to see regulation in the future, but [nonregulation] has allowed a lot of innovation in this space." He did add, however, that while he appreciates the creative freedom made possible by the lack of regulation,

> it doesn't necessarily provide the right guidance for what companies should be doing to constitute due diligence and

> research actually proving that the tools they're building work. So, we do take developing our tool set very seriously and want to make sure that it really adheres to what exactly a clinician would be using in their normal workflow. So, we're working with a research university on another study that will help prove efficacy of the tool set, and we'll continue to work with psychologists and psychiatrists as much as we can to make sure that what we're building really aligns with their tools as effectively as possible. . . . What we've created is absolutely a medical tool and, as we build off that tool set, we'll make sure that everything is super compliant. Just as we would something that's used in a typical healthcare setting.

Like Jordan, Levi predicted that FDA regulation of mental health applications is forthcoming, though he believes that for the moment "it would be irresponsible now to say [his application is] a medical device." In the future, however, he does

> plan to get FDA clearance. . . . We're going the way of the medical device, but right now the stress, anxiety world isn't heavily regulated and so that's allowed us to sort of, you know, get to market quickly and build the audience quickly. . . . So, when the FDA decides to regulate this industry, we'll be ready for it. . . . When we started this there weren't a ton of apps, and now there's a lot more apps. And so I think, you know, the best apps will rise to the top. But at the same time, I think regulation is going to help that too. So, I would not be surprised if more regulation was the way of the future, in that way.

Whereas Levi and Jordan's comments reflected a belief that nonregulation enhanced their abilities to be enterprising and creative, Mary spoke to ways in which a lack of oversight raises concerns related to data privacy and research ethics: "I'm in here doing science on the data [collected by the app] and nobody signed a consent form. They acknowledge the terms of service, which say, "Hey, we're probably going to analyze your data." But once it gets into [that] I'm looking at whether this works, it starts to feel like a clinical trial with no consent process." Consent to—or acknowledgment of—an application's Terms of Service or User Agreement is vastly different than consenting to participate in a research trial or having one's data studied. Yet Mary's sensitivity to this distinction was not voiced by other interviewees. Although it is possible that they did share those concerns, they may have been reluctant to tell me, as these disclosures might invite regulation by the FDA or other entity. I should emphasize the irony, however, in that while interviewees described their investments in creating technologies to improve the mental health of users, only Mary seemed to consider how psychologically devastating it would be to have one's mental-health-related privacy violated.

Advocates of mental health applications claim their existence facilitates the increased accessibility of mental healthcare services in that, by their very nature of being, they allow individuals to circumvent traditional medical industry models to obtain needed interventions. Yet as the industry fieldwork and interviews analyzed in this chapter reveal, accessibility as a construct is often considered and discussed only in relation to persons who already possess the requisite technologies that make downloading applications possible in the first place. The digital divide continues to be disregarded as somebody else's problem, despite many interviewees' claims that increasing access to mental healthcare is of the utmost concern to them.

Increasing the accessibility of mental healthcare services would seem, on its face, to be a priority for any person advocating for the implementation and use of mental health applications. Nonetheless pervasive slippages between the distinct notions of portability, accessibility, and usability throughout conversations with interviewees reflect a lack of differentiation between the varied meanings and significances of those terms. What's more, this also reflected lack of attunement to the possibility of diversity, including diverse needs, among persons who might benefit from mental health apps. Identity is multifaceted and complex, as are our subjectivities and positionalities. To overlook or ignore identity in relation to how it might affect accessing and obtaining the technologies through which mental health interventions are offered itself disregards long-standing inequities that are reflected and perpetuated by the digital divide. Accessibility is a multidimensional construct, and one that necessitates consideration of equity as well as the mere availability of services.[41] If there is not equitable distribution of—or access to—the technologies through which mental health interventions (including applications) are available, then we should not consider ourselves successful in increasing access to health interventions. Instead, we have only improved the continuum of mental healthcare services that were already available, and likely used by, those populations and persons who already reap the benefits of privileged subjectivities in the first place.

To that effect, consider that when I asked interviewees about the demographics of mental health application users, I was told that information collected about power users informs the development of strategies used to market toward the same population more effectively. This was contrary to how I had hoped demographic information might be used: to ascertain how mental health applications can be made more readily accessible and usable for persons beyond those who qualify as power users (who, to reiterate, are white, female, and young). Inaction in this regard perpetuates the methodical exclusion of nonwhite, nonfemale bodies from the technological imaginary that is referenced and used in conceptualizing who can benefit from mental health applications. We should understand these decisions, inadvertent or not, as reflective of attitudes and beliefs about whose bodies and mental health matter, and how certain bodies and identities continue to be privileged in our world more generally. These applications, in sum, are not created with the intent to improve the mental health of populations that continue to be underserved in matters of mental health resources and outcomes. That is what "increasing access" would truly entail. Rather, they are meant to improve the continuum of care for the same population (white women) that are already shown to consistently receive the most mental healthcare services of any population in the United States.

Taken together, this is emblematic of white prototypicality[42] across technological domains. Without intentional efforts to be actively inclusive and to consider how technologies can perpetuate marginalization, even inadvertently, it is unlikely that white prototypicality will ever be eliminated. Yet even this might not be enough, as capitalism and white prototypicality work hand-in-hand. Jason Mars, a computer science professor, once explained in an interview with the *New York Times* that although he identifies as African American, when his company created an application that involved a voice a deliberate choice was made to select one that sounded young, female, and white: "There's a kind of pressure to conform to the prejudices of the world. . . . It would be interesting to have a black guy [voice], but we don't want to create friction. . . . First we need to sell products."[43] Mars's comment suggests that if our primary concern is economic viability, then we must accept that Blackness, or that which might be interpreted as Black, is antithetical to profits. Until we are successful in abolishing the structures and systems that uphold racist and otherwise discriminatory beliefs and practices, even so simple an addition as including a "diverse" (i.e., nonwhite) sounding voice to a mental health application will likely never become the norm.

As Paul N. Edwards, one of the first scholars to highlight the political effects of computer systems, emphasized in the 1990s, programming is "a major cultural practice, a large-scale social form that has created and reinforced modes of thinking, systems of interaction, and ideologies of social control."[44] Discriminatory and prejudiced logics that manifest in technologies, including those embedded in mental health applications, trickle out into the "real" world, reifying biases and prejudices that already pervade social structures and systems. Revolutionizing dominant conceptualizations of whose bodies and lives matter is a prerequisite for revolutionizing access to healthcare technologies, and to claim that mental health applications are already doing so merely by existing is demonstrably unfounded. These tools are not increasing access; they are perpetuating the hegemony of whiteness and white supremacy.

Perhaps it is arguable that to *not* see oneself represented in these technologies, either through aural or visual content, is to the excluded population's betterment. By extension, the argument would go, we should worry more about those to whom these technologies do speak than those whom they do not speak. This, however, is a false choice. We need not pick only one or the other. We can be concerned both about who these applications systematically exclude as well as the new modalities of labor that others are tasked with as part of demonstrating their neoliberal citizenship. Just as significant as noting the burden of increased responsibilization upon some bodies and identities, we must simultaneously note those for whom participation in these regimes is neither expected nor even desired. Not only are they excluded from a technological imaginary; they are excluded from our social imaginary.

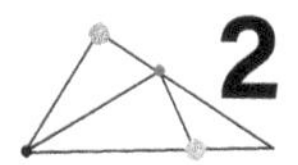

2

Psychosurveillance

> Facebook recently announced that it will expand, worldwide, a program designed to prevent suicide. The move comes after successful tests in the US to identify Facebook users who may be at risk. . . .
>
> Facebook began testing the software in March 2017, and while the company hasn't revealed full details about how the program works, we do know that the system relies on a pattern-matching algorithm. The program scans the text of Facebook posts and comments for certain phrases that could be signs of an impending suicide, like a friend commenting, "Are you okay?" or "Can I help?"
>
> If the software identifies a possible suicide threat, it's sent for review to a team of Facebook specialists trained in handling suicide and self-harm concern. Facebook also uses that pattern recognition to help escalate the most concerning reports, those of people who might need immediate attention. Those reports are escalated to local authorities, twice as quickly. In the past few months Facebook has worked with first responders on more than one hundred wellness checks based on this system, the company says. . . .
>
> Of course, machines can never replace psychological help or support systems for those in need. But when it comes to in-the-moment suicide prevention, another first responder could be the algorithm.[1]

In January 2018 *NBC News* uploaded a video to its website as part of a series titled *Algorithmics,* which sought to explore "how invisible, computer-controlled database sets of rules are making decisions for us, every day."[2] That month's feature, transcribed above, was titled "A Facebook Algorithm That's Designed for Suicide Prevention." Throughout the two-minute segment a male voice narrated as cartoon images of social media widgets, maps of the world, data sets, first responders, Facebook comments, Google searches, and more moved across the screen, meant to visually demonstrate the life-saving abilities of Facebook's latest algorithm.

Yet while the video provided a succinct summation of over a decade's worth of technological advances that made internet-based suicide and self-harm interventions possible, it omitted discussions of the broader-scale shifts in popular beliefs related to the areas of surveillance, technology, and mental health that facilitated acceptance of Facebook's algorithmic intervention in the first place. This chapter fills that void by identifying a practice and ethos that I term *psychosurveillance,* which refers to the monitoring of others' mental states online and represents a new dimension of responsibilization practices in line with neoliberalism's ongoing expansion. Unlike the previous chapter, which examined smartphone applications as one of governmentality's multiform tactics, psychosurveillance is an other-oriented modality that appeals to a communitarian—though still thoroughly neoliberal—spirit. Yet those communitarian appeals that are utilized by psychosurveillance's advocates mask psychosurveillance's propensity for exploitative labor practices. Their framing of psychosurveillance, as both altruistic and communitarian, foregrounds concern with others' mental states, and systematically disregards interest in the problematic labor that makes psychosurveillance possible.

This chapter begins by explaining the emergence and evolution of psychosurveillance, particularly how popular beliefs about the intersections of responsibilization, mental healthiness, and technology evolved during the early 2000s. I then discuss how psychosurveillance came to be articulated as a necessary element of responsible internet-based practices today. This includes an explanation of psychosurveillance's pedagogical function in the context of Facebook as well as its devaluation as a form of labor, demonstrated by further analyses of the platforms 7 Cups of Tea and Crisis Text Line. These case studies, taken together, demonstrate the interconnectedness of technologically facilitated surveillance with exploitative labor practices, and highlight the extent to which communitarian appeals obfuscate the negative effects of participating in regimes of psychosurveillance.

Psychosurveillance Begins

In 2008 Abraham Biggs, a nineteen-year-old from Pembroke Pines, Florida, became the first known person to livestream their suicide, doing so on the website Justin.tv.[3] Following his death social media strategist David Griner espoused a particularly significant sentiment when he claimed, "It's impossible for sites like Justin.tv to monitor everything that's going on, so that puts the burden on the community to help stop bad things from happening."[4] Griner's comment seemed to suggest that, if there was fault or blame to be placed for Biggs's death, it should fall upon those who had interacted with him on the internet. They were the ones who should have noticed that he was experiencing mental distress, and failed Biggs by missing whatever warning signs he had shared with them, indicative of his intent to end his life, beforehand. The aftermath of Biggs's death, therefore, should be understood as a pivotal moment. Not only did it mark a significant change in popular thinking and practices related to mental health surveillance on the internet, it generated an explicit directive as to who should be held responsible when those surveillance and monitoring practices fail: one's peers.

Van Houdt and Schinkel define communitarianism as "a paradoxical combination of neoliberalism with certain communitarian values."[5] Although neoliberalism emphasizes individual responsibilization, communitarianism emphasizes community-oriented responsibility. Communitarianism, including communitarian surveillance, operates in tandem with neoliberal sentiments and practices. Just as the diminishment of State responsibility reflects neoliberalism's expansion, in its place we see the rise of communitarianism, wherein we accept responsibility, not only for ourselves, but also for others in our networks and communities. Yet communitarianism's intersections with datafication, wherein behaviors and actions can be tracked and analyzed for predictive purposes,[6] have also facilitated our acceptance of widespread, technologically enabled surveillance.

Surveillance studies, as they have come to be called, owe much to Jeremy Bentham's writing about the panopticon: an architectural structure, a prison, that enables perpetual surveillance of prisoners.[7] Its design involves a central tower, located in the middle of a circular building, the interior-facing walls of which contain large windows. Those windows allow a guard who is located in the tower to watch inmates, but bright lights emanating from the tower and shining into the prisoners' cells prevent inmates from being able to see if or when the guard is present and watching them. The effects of the panopticon's design are multifold, as they facilitate "the omnipresence of the inspector . . . universal visibility of objects of surveillance; and third, the assumption of constant observation by the watched."[8]

Michel Foucault, in his own writings about the panopticon, suggested that the mere possibility of being subjected to surveillance explains why even those of us who are not prisoners, and are seemingly free, learn to moderate our conduct and behave as though we might be watched at all times.[9] Today this possibility of perpetual surveillance represents one of governmentality's multiform tactics, for just as the prisoners in Bentham's panopticon learned to moderate their behavior, so too do those of us utilizing an array of new technologies that are capable of tracking—or otherwise watching—us. Contemporary scholars, articulating these effects as panopticism, have utilized this framework in their analyses of an array of surveillance technologies, including hidden cameras,[10] social media platforms,[11] wearable technologies,[12] and more.

Psychosurveillance also draws upon Marc Andrejevic's conceptualization of *lateral surveillance*, a form of watching "that includes [people] keeping an eye on those around them."[13] Whereas surveillance discourses (including those of the panopticon) are often invoked to reflect power inequities between the "watcher" and "watchee," lateral surveillance draws our attention to the possibilities of watching afforded by peer-to-peer surveillance. However, as Andrejevic also notes, the "defining irony of the interactive economy is that the labor of detailed information gathering and comprehensive monitoring is being offloaded onto consumers in the name of their empowerment."[14] That we could come to believe that technology empowers us to prevent suicide, self-harm, or violence may seem an improbable leap. Yet as psychosurveillance exists along a spectrum of neoliberal responsibilization activities, there is nothing unbelievable about it. In our haste to applaud technological innovations, we forget to consider not only how innovations reflect our values and norms but also the roles they play in shaping them. Psychosurveillance, reflecting the belief that technology empowers us to save each other's lives, is therefore not really so improbable after all.

Empowerment through Watching (and Flagging)

Others have previously provided thorough analyses and critiques of commercial content moderation practices.[15] Much has been written, for example, about Facebook's mishandling of content moderation, particularly the significant emotional distress experienced by persons hired to provide those services. These moderators have claimed that their work, which includes viewing videos and images of child and animal abuse, pornography, hate speech, and violence, causes the development of PTSD, mental disorders, and facilitates otherwise unhealthy coping mechanisms.[16] In May 2020 Facebook ultimately settled a class-action lawsuit, paying $52 million to thousands of content moderators, despite never admitting to wrongdoing.[17] Yet psychosurveillance is vastly different from commercial content moderation in that it is framed as a form of volunteerism and, as such, does not require payment. Both are exploitative, but only the latter is framed as inherently undeserving of monetary compensation.

This results from psychosurveillance's relationship to *flagging*, a method of reporting content on internet platforms that is framed as a communitarian responsibility. As an act, flagging is "a mechanism for reporting offensive content . . . found on nearly all sites that host user-generated content . . . as well as in the comments sections on most blogs and news sites."[18] Yet flagging is not merely about the act of reporting, but also what reporting represents, as flags are "mechanisms [that] allow users to express their concerns within the predetermined rubric of a platform's 'community guidelines.'"[19]

Understandings of what constitute community violations vary across media platforms, between individuals who flag content, and by those who enforce content moderation policies. Consider, for example, the debate that ensued when the award-winning photograph titled "Terror of War," often referred to as the "Napalm Girl," was banned from Facebook. Despite its historical significance and notoriety, Facebook's content moderators believed that users' flagging of the image was justified: the image included a naked child, and in their view, this rendered it pornographic. After extensive public outcry, however, Facebook reconsidered its position and allowed the photograph to be reinstated on the website.[20] Although debate about what constitutes pornographic or otherwise "indecent" (that is, flaggable) content on social media platforms persists,[21] there is widespread agreement that any indication of intent to self-harm should always be reported, not because it is indecent, but because of our shared responsibility to intervene when we see that others are experiencing mental distress. Whereas the more generalized reporting of troubling content might "act as a mechanism to elicit and distribute user labor—users as a volunteer corps of regulators,"[22] psychosurveillance asks its "volunteer corps" to engage in surveillance with an eye only to matters of mental health and distress. To that effect the National Suicide Prevention Lifeline is proud of its collaborations with social networking websites and provides detailed instructions for reporting content on the platforms of Facebook, Twitter, Instagram, Snapchat, YouTube, and Periscope.[23]

In 2015 Facebook debuted new features that made the practice of psychosurveillance easier by including the option to report content indicating intent to self-harm.[24] An update from the company at the time emphasized that "keeping [users] safe is our most important responsibility," and added that if any Facebook user "sees a direct threat of suicide, we ask that they contact their local emergency services immediately. We also ask them to report any troubling content to us."[25] In 2017, however, things seemingly changed when Facebook celebrated the launch of its algorithmic intervention in suicide prevention, described in this chapter's opening. Upon its release Facebook's founder, Mark Zuckerberg, emphasized both the novelty and value of the algorithm:

> Starting today we're upgrading our AI tools to identify when someone is expressing thoughts about suicide on Facebook so we can help get them the support they need quickly. In the last month alone, these AI tools have helped us connect with first responders quickly more than 100 times. With all the fear about how AI may be harmful in the future, it's good to remind ourselves how AI is actually helping save people's lives today. There's a lot more we can do to improve this further. Today, these AI tools mostly use pattern recognition to identify signals—like comments asking if someone is okay—and then quickly report them to our teams working 24/7 around the world to get people help within minutes. In the future, AI will be able to understand more of the subtle nuances of language, and will be able to identify different issues beyond suicide as well, including quickly spotting more kinds of bullying and hate. Suicide is one of the leading causes of death for young people, and this is a new approach to prevention. We're going to keep working closely with our partners at Save.org, National Suicide Prevention Lifeline '1-800-273-TALK (8255)', Forefront Suicide Prevent, and with first responders to keep improving. If we can use AI to help people be there for their family and friends, that's an important and positive step forward.[26]

Facebook's algorithm is troubling for reasons beyond its perpetuation of techno-solutionism. Additionally, its implementation reveals that algorithms, even those used by social media platforms, are capable of independently manufacturing medical information about us. This algorithm, for example, analyzes every uploaded post to the Facebook platform, and scores them on a scale used to reflect the user's likelihood of causing "imminent harm."[27] Yet that information is not governed by data protection laws, nor is it HIPAA compliant, which is particularly worrisome in the context of Facebook's well-known history of data breaches.[28] John Torous, director of the digital psychiatry division at Boston's Beth Israel Deaconess Medical Center, has gone so far as to describe Facebook's algorithm as a form of "black box medicine."[29] Although algorithms and machine-learning processes are increasingly integrated into normative medical practice, debates are ongoing as to whether physicians and medical professionals ought to accept the black box nature of those interventions or whether they should demand access to their inner workings.[30] In the context of Facebook's algorithm, there is no clear demarcation between what constitutes the "medical" and the "social" when an algorithm itself is capable of transforming any and all user data through a technomedical gaze.

Nonetheless, once Facebook's public position became that an algorithm could prevent suicide, it should have seemingly eliminated the need for psychosurveillance. If a technology's capabilities surpass those of humans, which is what Zuckerberg's framing of the algorithm implied, then the work of human laborers would be rendered unnecessary and obsolete. This position was not altogether surprising, as Zuckerberg soon thereafter testified to a congressional panel his belief that AI is capable of solving a number of social problems.[31] Yet, in truth, there was no shift away from psychosurveillance—a human-generated form of labor—on Facebook following the algorithm's release, and a disparity manifested between what Zuckerberg publicly said about the algorithm and what the company's internal practices and policies remained. Through examination of that incongruity, evidenced by company documents that are discussed at length below, it becomes evident that psychosurveillance is still very much crucial to the platform's functioning. By extension, its reliance upon exploitative and dangerous labor practices also persists.

Consider Facebook's practices and policies in the context of livestreams, broadcasts that users can initiate at any time and from any location so long as they have an internet connection. Just as status updates and other posted content can be reported on Facebook due to perceived intent to self-harm, so too can livestreams. The experiences of filing a report on a livestream, and of having one's livestream reported, are as follows.[32] First, when an individual attempts to report a livestream, a window appears that asks why they are motivated to do so. "What's Going On?," they are asked, and can choose from a list of predetermined options, including violence, bullying, harassment, suicide or self-injury, nudity or sex acts, spam or scam, hate speech, unauthorized sales, or opt for the category of "other." If the suicide or self-harm option is selected, another screen pops up titled "What to do if a friend needs support." The following message then appears: "You reported [username's] post for suicide or self-injury. We'll take a look and have resources to send if [she/he] needs support. If you're concerned and not sure what else to do, read the resources we put together for guidance." If users choose to see those resources, they are brought to a screen with options to learn how to better support their friend, find a helpline's contact information, or connect with another Facebook friend (who, presumably, also knows the individual in distress).

The experience of being reported upon is entirely different. As the livestream broadcasts, because another user has flagged for reasons related to suicide or self-harm, a message is superimposed on the screen that is visible only to the individual who is broadcasting: "[Name], we're reaching out to offer help. Someone thinks you might need extra support right now and asked us to help." The broadcaster can then choose between a "CANCEL" option or "SEE RESOURCES." If the latter is selected, they are brought to another screen with the options of information to contact a helpline, see some tips, or talk with a friend. Facebook's motivations for this policy were articulated in March 2017 by the company's lead researcher in suicide prevention, Jennifer Guadagno. In a *New York Post* article, she emphasized that Facebook allows livestreams to continue, even when users are threatening suicide or engaging in self-harm. This course of action, Guadagno stated, "opens up the opportunity for people to reach out for support and for people to give support at this time that's critically important."[33]

All of this, however, should be considered alongside internal Facebook documents that were leaked and published by *The Guardian* in 2018. Those documents demonstrated that the company had motivations other than allowing "people to reach out for support," as Guadagno had claimed, when it adopted the policy of not interrupting livestreams flagged for self-harm or suicide related content.[34] Rather, Facebook's rationale was that "videos of violent deaths, while marked as disturbing, do not always have to be deleted because they can help create awareness of issues such as mental illness."[35] This reflects the pedagogical function of viewing livestreams and content depicting psychological distress: they teach Facebook users how to improve their own capacities as providers of psychosurveillance.

Elsewhere the same documents revealed that livestreamed content depicting self-harm would only be removed from Facebook "'once there's no longer an opportunity to help the person'—unless the incident is particularly newsworthy."[36] Despite the implementation of the algorithm, Facebook's priority remained to encourage psychosurveillance, and not to take preventative measures that would ensure the well-being of persons providing surveillance of others' mental states. If Facebook's desire was to prevent suicide, self-harm, and distress from exposure to that content, then allowing such livestreams would, in fact, be antithetical to that goal. Ample research has established that high-profile suicides may lead to copycat behaviors, a phenomenon known as the Werther effect.[37] Therefore Facebook's decision to keep livestreams accessible, even when they depict self-harm, suicide, or otherwise "particularly newsworthy" persons or events, is rendered even more suspect by the possibility of that content triggering suicide contagion.[38]

Facebook's prioritization of the pedagogical function of mental distress (that is, its presumed ability to enhance psychosurveillance practices) endangers its users. It is irresponsible and cruel to allow livestreams to continue, or remain accessible, knowing full well that they might facilitate mental distress among other users who "watch" their peers self-harm. Regardless, the Facebook company's framing of psychosurveillance as integral to community building reflects the ways in which responsibilization and risk taking are increasingly considered part of normative practices, even when doing so risks the health and safety of the community at large.

7 Cups of Tea and Psychosurveillance's Devaluation

Facebook's mission is "to give people the power to build community . . . to stay connected with friends and family, to discover what's going on in the world and to share and express what matters to them."[39] Psychosurveillance, while part of what is involved in the formation of—and participation in—that community, is not its be-all and end-all. Yet there are other platforms and services predicated entirely upon psychosurveillance, due to its presumed ability to generate social bonds and form communities. In such cases, "community" is formed not only by those who are willing to undergo psychosurveillance as its subjects, but also by those willing to provide the labor that is integral to psychosurveillance.

Research demonstrates that individuals with mental illnesses benefit from social connections that are often found in supportive online communities.[40] As such, there are many platforms, available as smartphone applications and internet websites, which enable users to connect with others and communicate about their experiences with mental illness and distress. 7 Cups of Tea is one such platform, both a website and smartphone application, that I analyzed over a number of months as I conducted this research. Initially I perused its offerings, though later I began to work as a Listener, a designated volunteer whose role is to message with other users experiencing varying levels of mental distress.

Unlike platforms that connect persons experiencing distress with paid-for services from licensed mental health professionals, 7 Cups offers to provide human-to-human connections for free. "We live in a world where you can be surrounded by people, but still feel lonely, with nobody to turn to when things get rough," the 7 Cups homepage reads.

> But being heard is an important part of being human. Psychologist, Glen Moriarty saw that there was great power in listening, but he knew not everyone had someone to talk to. He started to wonder. "How can I make being heard a reality for everyone?"
>
> *That's why 7 Cups was born.*
>
> Thanks to thousands of volunteer listeners stepping up to lend a friendly ear, 7 Cups is happy to say, "We're here for you!"
>
> No matter who you are or what you're going through, this is a place where you'll be heard and cared for. We might be strangers on the surface, but underneath we're just the friends you haven't met yet.[41]

7 Cups' Listeners, the unpaid volunteers who make it possible to be "heard," are told that their work has "the power to change lives."[42] Yet again, Listeners are not trained mental health professionals. They are simply persons who, for whatever reason, are willing to spend time messaging with anonymous others on the platform. 7 Cups of Tea does also offer to connect users with trained mental health professionals but, unlike communicating with Listeners, there are fees associated with those sessions. Nonetheless, some research that is available on the platform's website suggests that 7 Cups has potentially therapeutic benefits, even solely as a result of messaging with Listeners.[43]

Unlike the ways in which Facebook's (or other social media platforms') users might unintentionally stumble upon flag-worthy content, report it, and then return to life as usual, persons who come to 7 Cups of Tea are utilizing the technology for the sole purpose of psychosurveillance. They are either submitting themselves to the surveillance regimes provided by Listeners, or they are surveilling other users while acting as Listeners themselves. Yet because Listening is framed by 7 Cups as a form of altruistic volunteerism, it is also highly devalued. This results in a paradox. On the one hand, Listeners push the boundaries of neoliberal responsibilization by working in ways that seemingly demonstrate that individualized, privatized solutions to mental distress are possible. Yet on the other, as my own experiences as a Listener illustrate, they are in no way capable of adequately responding to the mental distress experienced by those with whom they communicate. This makes the work of Listening dangerous. Not only are Listeners encouraged to believe that we are responsible for improving the mental health of others, although we are fundamentally unequipped to do so, we are also apt to experience significant psychological distress as a result of our failures in this work.

Although 7 Cups' Listeners are not mental health professionals, they do receive training from the platform itself. I underwent that training, which began with the following message:

> Active listening is a great way to care and support another person. At first, you will likely find it to be a bit challenging. In normal relationships, we tend to take turns talking and

> sharing. With active listening, you are focused primarily on the other person. Your careful listening helps the other person to feel heard, valued, and understood. Keep in mind that active listening is not counseling or advice giving. You shouldn't try to solve their problems.[44]

Training involved a short, online course during which I—a Listener-to-be—was taught to reflect emotions via online messaging, to ask questions of those with whom I would chat, to evaluate and improve my listening skills, to engage in active listening, to maintain the confidentiality of those with whom I messaged, to learn when to suggest that users engage with 7 Cups of Tea's trained mental health professionals, to discern trolls from persons experiencing genuine distress, and to practice internet safety. Yet all of this training took no more than ten minutes. While my own background is devoid of clinical experience, it does not require an advanced degree to know that in the context of working with persons experiencing psychological distress, ten minutes of preparation is woefully inadequate. I even found it frightening, not only because of how inadequate *I* felt about *myself* as a prospective caregiver to others over this platform, but in that I could imagine other Listeners taking the training even *less* seriously, providing *worse* care and, potentially, causing harm to those with whom they would interact.

I surmise that one of the internal justifications for the limited scope of Listener training results from assumptions about Listeners themselves: that we come to the 7 Cups platform already knowledgeable about mental illness and distress. As psychologist Otto Wahl suggests, mental illness has become "a topic about which most laypersons know a little but few know a lot."[45] This familiarity might be attributed to the increasing frequency with which mental distress and disorders are represented in media and popular discourse, the positive effects of destigmatization campaigns,[46] or our own lived experiences. It also reflects what Nikolas Rose describes as the dispersion of the "psy" in popular culture: "the heterogeneous knowledges, forms of authority and practical techniques that constitute psychological expertise."[47] None of this, however, qualifies one to competently assess others' mental states, or to provide help in times of crisis, even in combination with ten minutes of Listener training.

Despite my trepidations, after completing the training I scheduled a block of time during which I would volunteer. I was then brought to my Listener home page. There I had the option to customize my profile and access charts that would, one day, come to reflect the amount of time I had volunteered as a Listener. At the bottom of the page a colored bar showed the number of 7 Cups users who were waiting for Listeners to converse with them. If the bar was green, I realized, it meant that an "acceptable" number of users were waiting. Conversely an orange or red colored bar meant that there were too many waiting for help and I—and the other Listeners—needed to initiate conversations with them more quickly.

On this, my first day of Listening, the bar was green, and I therefore felt comfortable taking some time to explore the pending conversation requests and consider users' reasons for wanting to talk. I clicked on a window titled General Conversation Requests. "General requests go out to *ALL LISTENERS*" it read. "Please *SELECT REQUESTS FROM THE TOP* or topics that you care about. Thank you! Current user wait time average 2 Minute(s) / 9 Second(s)." Of the six users waiting to chat, two had not specified their reasons for wanting to communicate with Listeners. The other four, however, had done so, and their reasons appeared below their usernames. One had written "Depression" and another had chosen "Managing Emotions." A third opted for "Breakups" and a fourth was "General Mental Illness." Although I assume that 7 Cups of Tea's creators felt that Listener training would prepare us for all conversational topics, I still believed that messaging about diagnosed mental illness and disorders was beyond the scope of what I ethically should do. I therefore chose to converse with the user who had indicated they wanted to talk about breakups.

As someone who has initiated breakups, been on the receiving end of breakups, and seen and heard about friends', celebrities', and family members' breakups, I did not anticipate that this would be a particularly challenging conversation. Yet this assumption proved to be entirely incorrect. The window that popped up on my screen when I clicked on that user's Listener request foreshadowed what was to come. "Care for Yourself First," that message read:

> We all want to care for others, but we can only adequately care for other people if we are in good shape ourselves. If we are not in good shape, then we run the risk of hurting ourselves, others, and burning out. Take good care of ourselves means eating, exercising, and sleeping well. We care for you and want you to rest and take care of yourself. You matter and are important to us!

Before I could send a welcome message or greeting to the other user, they began to send me information about how they were feeling, using a rating scale that I believe was suggested to them by the 7 Cups of Tea platform:

> THEM: I am this challenged (1–10): 10
>
> THEM: I feel this way this often (days): Everyday

During the course of all communications the 7 Cups of Tea platform offered suggestions for what I, as a Listener, should not only say, but also when to say it. For example, when this person shared that they felt this way "Everyday," a "Listener Tip" popped up on screen with the following: "Next say (or copy and paste) "If you are feeling like you need expert guidance, then I'd recommend talking with a therapist. . . . If I feel like you'd be better served by a therapist, then I might make a referral later on in our conversation." Although I opted to ignore most Listener Tips, they are included in the following transcripts at the points in which they appeared.

> THEM: I've felt this way for this long: Since the past week
>
> THEM: The love of my life left me yesterday

During all of this, along the left side of the screen was a reminder visible to me that, if this person needed more help than I could offer, I should click to offer them 7 Cup's therapy services.

ME: Is there anything that I can talk to you about? Or maybe, if you want advice, would you like some resource referrals?

THEM: I need help.

Listener Tip: Relate to this member as you would a good friend and simply care for them. That is the most powerful thing you can do.

THEM: She is the love of my life.

THEM: She just up and left suddenly.

Listener Tip: Say things like "Oh okay" or "I understand" or "mhmmm" to show that you are paying attention and listening. Avoid chatspeak or deliberate misspellings of words. Please use full words, not abbreviations.

THEM: She said she stopped loving me.

ME: I am so sorry that happened.

Listener Tip: Reflect back to the member summarizing what the member is saying. It is okay to use their same or similar words. Summarize throughout the conversation.

The conversation quickly became much more difficult than I had anticipated. Although I knew that we would be talking about breakups, I had thought it would be more along the lines of a philosophical discussion. Maybe this person was sad about a recent breakup, I had imagined, or was feeling a little lonely after a breakup. In retrospect I suppose it was naïve to not realize that only significant distress would lead an individual to want to talk about losing the love of their life with me, a stranger, on the internet.

I felt powerless throughout our communications, as I had been trained not to respond to this person as a friend might have. During the course of a normal conversation about a breakup I might ask for details, provide comfort, read nonverbal cues, and assess how they were feeling more comprehensively. Yet in an online context, wherein my role was to provide active listening based solely upon typed information, and not to ask the questions that a genuine friend might, none of that was possible. According to my training, pressing for details was beyond the scope of what a

Listener should do. My role was only to reflect others' feelings and statements back to them in hopes that that would help them heal. Yet the more I messaged with this person the clearer it became that I would be unable to alleviate their distress.

ME: You said that you need help? What can I help you with?

THEM: I'm terribly depressed.

THEM: I find myself bursting into tears randomly.

In my training I had been told that if an individual indicates that they might be suicidal I should provide them with the National Suicide Prevention Lifeline's contact information. Yet this person, while stating that they were depressed (without clarifying whether they felt depressed or were diagnosed with depression), had not indicated intent to self-harm. Therefore, according to my 7 Cups training, I should have been able to help them, and despite my genuine desire and attempts to do so, I seemed to be failing. Although I felt guilty, as though it was due to my own incompetency as a Listener, I came to the conclusion that this person needed the help of a mental health professional. I relayed to them that in my (limited) capacity as a Listener I could not provide much help, but if they were open to it, I would share information about 7 Cups of Tea's therapy services:

ME: Hm, you think you are depressed? And are crying a lot?

ME: It might be helpful for you to talk to someone who is a professional, who can actually provide you with advice and help. Unfortunately I am just a listener and not a trained mental health professional.

ME: Can I provide you with information about resources that you might find more helpful?

Listener Tip: We'll teach you many new skills to help you grow both personally and professionally. 7 Cups is a safe place to learn and grow.

THEM: Please do.

I was relieved that they accepted my offer and clicked a link on the left side of the page that automatically pasted referral information into our chat box. I modified its text to fit more naturally into our conversation.

ME: I am happy to keep chatting with you, but I would recommend that you also check out our 7 Cups therapists here: 7cups.com/online-therapy

Listener Tip: When you show compassion to others, you also learn to show compassion to yourself. You will think to yourself, "Wait a second, I was just really loving to that person. I'm going to show myself that same level of love and compassion."

THEM: Okay thank you

ME: You are so welcome. Please check in with me again any time.

Listener Tip: Blocking a guest is appropriate when they are being abusive, sexting, or insulting. It is not appropriate when you simply do not approve of the issue the person is struggling with. If you are triggered, let the member know that they need to connect with another Listener because you are not the best fit to address this issue.

I do not possess the professional training or skills to dissociate myself from the mental and emotional distress of others, nor do I know whether persons are prone to exaggerate their feelings of distress on the internet or platforms such as 7 Cups of Tea. But as my very first experiences as a Listener progressed, and as I ruminated over those experiences after signing out of the platform, my own anxieties and fears amplified. My hands were sweating, my heartbeat felt palpable in my chest, and my mind raced. I had been the perfect neoliberal citizen, volunteering my time to provide psychosurveillance to the betterment of others and the community. Seemingly I had been successful, as I had discerned that this individual needed more help than I could provide, and at my suggestion they had agreed to work with a mental health professional. Yet, despite all of these "successes," I was now experiencing psychological distress myself. I felt nervous and anxious, revisiting and replaying our conversation in my head, and wondering if I had said and done all of the right things. *What if I hadn't?*, I wondered. *What were the stakes? What if this person had not followed up with an actual mental health professional, had been experiencing mental distress far more severe that I had been able to discern, and had harmed themselves or someone else?* I know that I could have left our conversation at any time. Perhaps, then, I would not have felt so distraught in its aftermath. Yet my fear had been that exiting prematurely might exacerbate the other person's mental distress, which would make me truly culpable not only for their well-being but also any harm they might have inflicted upon themself or others.

A few hours after that conversation, however, my concerns became somewhat alleviated. I received an email from 7 Cups of Tea informing me the person with whom I had been messaging had taken the time to "rate" my skills as a Listener. They had designated me four of a possible five stars. I was surprised. I had not realized that the work of Listening would ever be framed as so explicitly transactional. Despite the platform's insistence that my work was invaluable and life changing, here I was being provided with a quantitative evaluation of my work. Yet the rating system was not reciprocal. I could not provide any concrete evaluation of this other user, even if only in order to pass information on to the mental health professional with whom I hoped they had followed up. I admit that, in addition to being shocked that I was rated at all, I was also miffed that my rating hadn't been higher. Nonetheless, I found solace in the fact that this user was willing to rate me, as someone experiencing severe emotional distress probably would not have been motivated to do so.[48]

I volunteered as a Listener for 7 Cups of Tea on a few more occasions, but it never became something I enjoyed. I rarely felt that I was providing adequate support for persons in need and, more often than not, the platform was deliberately misused by those who messaged with me. During one exchange I asked my conversational partner if there was anything in particular that they wanted to talk about. "As a Listener I can't give advice, but I can definitely listen," I told them. "No thanks," they responded. "I was hoping to find a normal person not some brainwashed rule obsessed goon[.]" The omnipresent anxiety that hovered over me when I volunteered as a Listener was, at the very least, alleviated when I received abusive messages such as this:

> THEM: hi, my cousin invited me to a frat party. i've never gone to one before and I was wondering if you have
>
> ME: Hi. I'm sorry I can't give advice or anything like that on this platform—as a Listener my role is to listen to anything you want to talk about.
>
> THEM: I'm a Listener too
>
> ME: Ok cool!
>
> THEM: i asked you a simple question
>
> THEM: but apparently that's too much for you to handle
>
> ME: I'm sorry you feel that way.
>
> ME: Do you have anything else you want to talk about?
>
> THEM: you should hear the choking sound of a baby as i shove my cock down its throat

I much preferred receiving vile, disgusting messages to the anxiety I experienced while wondering whether I was ever actually helping persons experiencing mental distress. Abuse proved much easier for me to emotionally detach from than the helplessness I experienced when I could do nothing for persons in pain. Once, for example, when I believed that someone with whom I messaged would benefit from talking to a real therapist, I asked whether they would like a referral to the 7 Cups of Tea mental health professionals. "They can help you more than I can," I explained.

> THEM: I can't spare any money for a therapist
>
> THEM: but thank you
>
> THEM: it's OK

Psychosurveillance on 7 Cups of Tea is markedly different than that which transpires on traditional social media platforms. In the context of Facebook, for example, users' identities are public, and psychosurveillance is a function secondary to maintaining social connections. 7 Cups of Tea, on the other hand, is a platform created for the sole purpose of finding support from others, and on which participants willingly becoming the subjects of psychosurveillance.

Listeners are intended to assess the level of distress of others despite having no formal training in any mental health field and no baseline knowledge about those with whom they communicate. Despite being told that their work is an altruistic form of volunteerism, their function is fundamentally an economic one. Devoid of context and communication cues, those who work as Listeners are engaged in a high-stakes enterprise wherein their role is to determine who can be recruited for the platform's paid-for services. My responsibility in the 7 Cups of Tea ecosystem was not to help others so much as it was to evaluate their mental health. I was a mechanism of discernment, a replaceable cog tasked with differentiating between those whose communicative needs could be satisfied by having their words reflected back to them and those who might be willing to pay to work with 7 Cups of Tea's therapists. The benefit of volunteering as a Listener, I had been told, was that 7 Cups of Tea would teach me "many new skills. . . . 7 Cups is a safe place to learn and grow." Yet my role, in actuality, was to funnel users into a pay-to-play system after evaluating their needs and willingness to pay for services.

Crisis Text Line and Communitarianism

Crisis Text Line, a text-based service that allows persons to anonymously message with volunteers, was launched in August 2013. Nancy Lublin, then-CEO of DoSomething.org, realized there was a need for a text-message based service when a volunteer at DoSomething notified her of a series of alarming text messages wherein an anonymous sender disclosed being repeatedly raped by their father. Although the DoSomething volunteer encouraged that person to contact the Rape, Abuse & Incest National Network (RAINN), they felt that this recommendation was not enough. As a result, the volunteer began collaborating with Lublin on a project that came to fruition as Crisis Text Line.[49] To date over four million conversations have been held via the platform, with users from all fifty American states.[50]

Unlike the process of becoming a Listener on 7 Cups of Tea, volunteering for Crisis Text Line is much more rigorous, and requires thirty hours of training. Yet the appeals used to recruit volunteers for Crisis Text Line are similar to those of 7 Cups. Those benefits, as described on Crisis Text Line's website, include "an opportunity to hone your skills in communication, counseling, and intervention . . . which can in turn sharpen your crisis management skills! But most of all, you'll feel supported. This is a community. We are a big awesome family."[51] A number of blog posts written by volunteers themselves, wherein they describe and reflect upon the value of volunteering, are again like those of 7 Cups of Tea's Listeners: they feel positively transformed by this work, and enjoy contributing to their community.[52]

I contacted Crisis Text Line, hoping for an opportunity to discuss the platform and its volunteer program in more depth than what internet searches revealed. Elizabeth Sweezey Morrell, Crisis Text Line's recruitment and admissions manager, responded to my inquiry, and we were able to have a discussion on the phone. She described volunteers as "more women than men" and also "more East Coast than other time zones, more twenties and thirties than sixties and seventies, more white than other races, and we don't ask for income, though most of our volunteer have college degrees." When I brought up the fact that Crisis Text Line struggles to retain volunteers, despite the accolades it receives and the perceived benefits of volunteering,[53] Morrell reframed the problem more optimistically. She noted that although not everyone continues to volunteer for the platform indefinitely, they have "trained about 20,000 people, and all of those people have helped someone in crisis."

Morrell also shared with me that Crisis Text Line had previously considered monetary compensation for volunteers, but currently offered only "incentives based on the number of conversations a Crisis Counselor has taken." This approach was in line with what Lublin had written in a blog post for Crisis Text Line's website in 2018:

> The best way to keep people involved . . . is to reward them. Show them how much you appreciate them. In order to do this, we created Levels. They're a huge source of pride for our Crisis Counselors, with each level corresponding to a certain number of conversations taken. Levels are a form of thanking our Crisis Counselors. It's an acknowledgment of amazing work completed. Personal milestones. They are self-paced, transparent, and available to everyone—just like levels of a game. We found that adding more levels and transparency has increased retention among our newer Crisis Counselors by 42%.[54]

Morrell described this to me as "gamification in the form of levels," and added that Crisis Text Line offers "something when [volunteers] hit each level—this could be a water bottle, T shirt, a redeemable promo or coupon, or some other surprise."

I then asked what reasons have been given, if any, by volunteers when they decide to stop working for the platform. Morrell responded that Crisis Text Line intentionally does not ask volunteers why they stop because they "don't want to induce guilt." She added, however, that of those who choose to disclose reasons for leaving, they "mention that it's difficult work emotionally and they need to take a break. Others share that they suffer from their own mental health issues and this is more triggering than they expected. Others have busy lives with family and/or work, or have things come up, and they have to step away or stop entirely."

Unlike what transpires in the context of the 7 Cups of Tea platform, where volunteers are framed as empathetic, listening ears, there are no attempts to deny the psychologically demanding nature of volunteering for Crisis Text Line. Even Morrell herself did not shy away from using the word "work" to describe all that volunteering entails. This may have been because Crisis Text Line does not provide any service that requires payment, unlike 7 Cups of Tea, which charges fees to connect persons with mental health professionals. Rather, volunteers themselves are the be-all and end-all of what Crisis Text Line provides. Without them and the labor they provide, there would be no Crisis Text Line.

Psychosurveillance constitutes not only an expansion of what we conceptualize as fitting in the realm of everyday knowledge (in this case, the ability to assess the mental healthiness of others), but also the ways in which neoliberalization necessitates new, technologically facilitated practices that are framed as integral to keeping our communities, loved ones, and ourselves, safe. This change is significant. Not long ago the ability to ascertain the mental healthiness or distress of others was considered possible only by those working in fields related to mental health. Now, however, due to the dispersion of the psy throughout popular culture, members of the general public have increasingly accepted that psychosurveillance is a necessary part of responsible citizenship practices.

Psychosurveillance's emergence and popularization result from a growing emphasis upon communitarian approaches to health interventions, even in the domain of mental health. Yet psychosurveillance would not have become possible without the prior normalization of peer-to-peer surveillance, which we were already largely desensitized to due to its centrality in social networking platforms. In lieu of finding structural solutions to the growing need for mental healthcare interventions, individual citizens are now encouraged to see *themselves* as the solutions to mental illnesses and others' experiences of mental distress. We are told that utilizing various technologies and platforms will empower us to change others' lives for the better, and that although this constitutes a form of work, the benefits of helping others outweigh whatever distress we might experience in the process.

Psychosurveillance involves a spectrum of practices that initially appear to be motivated by altruism and communitarianism, but which are in actuality the result of intersecting economic impetuses with responsibilization discourses. Those who provide the work of psychosurveillance add palpable economic and social value to the platforms on which they volunteer. Yet at the same time they are told that the "rewards" of doing so are intangible, though still valuable, in the forms of personal growth, feelings of pride and accomplishment, or perhaps (in the case of Crisis Text Line) as water bottles. These appeals of selflessness and altruism, of offering to help others in times of mental distress, are utilized to obscure psychosurveillance's propensity for exploiting its labor force.

My argument is not that financial payment is necessary to make psychosurveillance a fair exchange between workers and those who employ their services. Instead, my intent is to highlight the incongruity of for-profit entities devaluing the labor and risks of psychosurveillance while simultaneously perpetuating the belief that psychosurveillance is a necessary element of neoliberal citizenship and communitarianism. I am not suggesting that we should ignore the mental distress of others, even when that distress is evident to us only in digital spaces. Rather, I am emphasizing the inconsistency between framing content moderation as labor when we are also told that psychosurveillance is to be provided for free because it is a form of altruistic volunteerism. One necessitates payment; the other does not. Both involve risks for workers, yet only the latter gets away with utilizing appeals of personal growth in lieu of payment.

Although we so often conceptualize mental illness and distress as private, lonely, and isolating, psychosurveillance and the platforms on which it transpires create the possibility of communities and relationships existing regardless of geographic proximity and location. Yet alongside those possibilities, psychosurveillance nonetheless remains a high-risk form of labor. Not only is there a possibility of misinterpreting indicators of others' mental states, but also that persons engaged in the surveillance of others will experience mental distress themselves in the same way that paid content moderators have been known to do. Nonetheless, unpaid labor, even that which constitutes psychosurveillance, is an integral part of capitalist economies.[55] We are therefore unlikely to witness its disappearance any time in the near future.

Psychosurveillance reflects how an ethos of altruism itself can be transformed, and even warped, in the context of technologies and the practices they endeavor. In this case we see how self-sacrifice, the appropriation of psychological risks, and a willingness to work without compensation become not only normalized but also the accepted outcomes of wanting to help others. While

I am not arguing against volunteerism per se, I do take issue with encouraging nonexperts to appropriate risks (both to themselves and others) in domains where nonexpertise may result in harm. For so long as we continue to fetishize technologies, and to accept increased responsibilization even in realms where it is highly inappropriate and unjustified, this exploitation will persist.

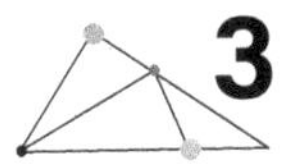

3

Chatbots and Therapeutic AI

Some of the oldest known imaginings about artificial life are found in ancient Greek mythology, demonstrating that humankind has been preoccupied with questions of what it might be like to live alongside those who are "made, not born," for millennia.[1] To that effect Adrienne Mayor, in the book *Gods and Robots: Myths, Machines, and Ancient Dreams of Technology,* suggests that the ancient "stories of Jason and the Argonauts, the bronze robot Talos, the techno-witch Medea, the genius craftsman Daedalus, the fire-bringer Prometheus, and Pandora, the evil fembot created by Hephaestus, the god of invention" reflect our enduring preoccupation with artificial life.[2] Yet unlike the ancient Greeks, today many of us interact with entities that are "made, not born," and do so on a regular basis. These encounters are so normative, in fact, that they are part of our daily routines: we scroll through our personalized viewing recommendations generated by Netflix,[3] look at suggested items when we shop online,[4] and listen and speak to the "virtual assistants" whose disembodied voices inhabit our smartphones.[5]

Despite being human-made and inorganic, it is possible for these entities to play important roles in shaping our beliefs, attitudes, and behaviors. That is why it is so problematic to believe that they are value neutral and apolitical when, in fact, the opposite is true. Even Netflix's algorithm has been shown to engage in racial profiling, altering films' promotional materials based upon its assumptions about account holders' ethnicities;[6] online shopping algorithms discriminate based on presumptions about race and gender;[7] and virtual assistants are more often unable to identify words and commands from people of color than those spoken by white users.[8] This is not to say that those responsible for these tool sets intentionally create technologies that are discriminatory, yet discriminatory practices are the outcome of their use nonetheless. Rather than focus upon the stated intention of a technology's creator(s), a more productive approach is to examine the social and cultural effects of a technology upon its implementation and use. While intentionality certainly matters, so too do the ways in which technologies replicate long-standing prejudices and beliefs, even unintentionally.

With that in mind, this chapter examines a particular technological form made possible by algorithms: artificially intelligent chatbots intended to improve the mental healthiness of their users. As I am unable to open these chatbots' "black boxes," the mode of analysis undertaken involves textual analysis, interviews, and autoethnography. I describe my experiences utilizing three popular therapeutic chatbots and also include information from discussions with two of those chatbots' creators.

Despite the pervasiveness of celebratory discourses that herald therapeutic chatbots as a potential solution to the ongoing mental health crisis,[9] this chapter demonstrates that they are neither feasible interventions nor useful for all populations equally. Similar to arguments presented in my analysis of smartphone applications, this genre of therapeutic technology encourages responsibilization practices only for a hegemonic user, imagined as white, and thereby perpetuates the systematic exclusion and erasure of other bodies and identities. Although these chatbots are incapable of expanding access to mental healthcare interventions, their social and cultural function remains significant. Not only do they read and understand their users in ways that reify white hegemony, they are similarly imbued with the markers and characteristics of whiteness themselves.

Discriminatory Health Technologies and Neoliberalism

On August 16, 2017, Chukwuemeka Afigbo uploaded a video to Twitter with the following caption: "If you have ever had a problem grasping the importance of diversity in tech and its impact on society, watch this video."[10] In the video we see what appears to be a white person's hand beneath a soap dispenser. A wad of soap is pumped onto its open palm. "Nice," says a voice off camera. The hand pulls away. A moment later a darker-skinned hand is also outstretched below the dispenser, just like the hand before it. Now, however, nothing happens. "Too black," voices murmur in the background. The hand keeps at it though, moving up and down at various speeds, attempting to make the dispenser work. Eventually the hand stops, grabs a white paper towel, and returns to the same spot beneath the dispenser. Now, with the white paper towel covering it, multiple pumps of soap are dispensed onto its palm. When the towel is removed again, however, and the uncovered, dark-skinned palm is beneath the machine, it no longer releases soap.

Afigbo's video went viral and debate ensued. Some viewers argued that the technology was racist because it had discriminated against darker-skinned users, evidenced by its "refusal" to provide them with soap.[11] Others, even on Afigbo's own Twitter page, declared that this was a mere technological error, not a manifestation or reflection of racism or racist beliefs. Still others investigated the origins of the soap dispenser, determining that the infrared technology it utilized to determine when hands were located beneath it was known to not work well (if at all) for nonwhite persons.[12]

I share the story of Afigbo's experience with the soap dispenser because of its relevance to broader debates about technological discrimination. Although some believe that we must find "evidence of racial [or otherwise discriminatory] thinking in design or deployment" before characterizing technologies as racist or perpetuating marginalization and oppression,[13] others argue that technologies inherently reflect the biases and prejudices of their creators, and that these discriminatory logics are sometimes only visible once those tools are used. Therefore, when a technology's creators endow it with the ability to only recognize the existence of a light-skinned or white body, as was the case with Afigbo's soap dispenser, that technology should be understood as perpetuating the marginalization of those whom it cannot recognize. They exist beyond its technological imaginary. This reflects Simone Browne's description of "prototypical whiteness" in technologies, wherein tools are created for imagined users who are presumably white.[14] White bodies are, in essence, most technologies' default bodies.

While it might seem inconsequential to discuss technology and race in the context of handwashing, we should not forget that handwashing is now, more than ever, a practice representative of "good" neoliberal citizenship. This became particularly evident during the spring of 2020, when the interconnectedness of washing one's hands with assuming responsibility for preventing the spread of COVID-19 became explicit in news and other media content.[15] Handwashing exists, therefore, along the same spectrum of health-related responsibilization practices as do mental health technologies. In an argument that parallels some of those that this book has previously made about the individuation of responsibility, others have suggested that "handwashing campaigns reinforce an individualistic model of public health, one premised to a significant extent on the necessity of behavior change rather than structural intervention."[16]

No matter, Afigbo's soap dispenser demonstrates an important distinction between matters of accessibility and usability. Afigbo and his cohort could easily *access* the soap dispenser. All they had to do was find their way to the washroom and extend their palms below it. The dispenser was not, however, *equally usable* by each person in the group. If there are certain bodies, groups, and identities that are unable to be seen by technology, literally unseen in the context of this soap dispenser, those persons are prohibited from participation in the practices that constitute good neoliberal citizenship. Although this book primarily makes those arguments in the context of mental health technologies, even a discriminatory soap dispenser can illustrate them.

Algorithms and AI in Medicine

Any introductory computer science textbook will provide a definition of "algorithm" that goes something like the following: algorithms are formulas, sequences of computer code, that generate automated responses to queries and range from simple to complex.[17] Similarly, "machine learning" is a phrase used to describe algorithms that are able to improve their performance in responding to tasks due to repeated experience executing them.[18] "Deep learning" algorithms, unlike simpler machine learning algorithms, are intended to function similarly to the multilayered, complex human brain. They are able to process data and information that is more abstract and rawer than what a machine learning program might do.[19] Regardless of whether they are complex, simple, or deep learning, algorithms are shrouded in mystery, as the technical dimensions of what make them function is often considered proprietary information. Yet as anthropologist Nick Seaver points out, in our analyses of algorithms we should not be "talking about algorithms in the technical sense," but rather pursuing understandings of the broader "algorithmic systems" to which they belong.[20] These systems involve more than code, additionally encompassing domains of the social, cultural, political, and, in the case of this book, the medical.

Algorithms are utilized in the creation of artificial intelligence (AI), although algorithms and AI are not one and the same. "Artificial intelligence" is used to describe actions or behaviors that appear intelligent and are performed by machines.[21] Yet they need only appear to possess intelligence because, at the time of writing at least, there is no such thing as an autonomously intelligent machine. Alan Turing noted this vital distinction in his conceptualization of an imitation game, which has come to act as a litmus test in determining whether a technology should be described as intelligent.[22] If a human evaluator cannot tell the difference between a machine and a human, Turing claimed, the technology has effectively passed the test and should be considered intelligent.

Turning back to Seaver's suggestion that we ought to conceptualize algorithms as not only code but also sociocultural forces that produce and reproduce power relations, we should consider as well the reasons that advocates of AI-based medical interventions are in favor of those approaches. Some, for example, believe that "medical AI demonstrate that the algorithms can do as well as (if not better than) expert human physicians in some fields of medical diagnosis and prognosis."[23] Others suggest that utilizing algorithmic decision-making in clinicians' workflows will not make human oversight or practitioners obsolete, but will instead extend and enhance their capabilities.[24] Yet the history of AI in medicine, which dates back to the 1960s,[25] shows that rather than serve a democratizing function, algorithms fundamentally reproduce inequities. During the 1970s, for example, St. George's Hospital Medical School in the United Kingdom began to utilize a computer program to help screen candidates for admission. Although that algorithm "mimicked the choices admission staff had made in the past," it ultimately "denied interviews to as many as 60 applicants because they were women or had non-European sounding names. The code wasn't the work of some nefarious programmer; instead, the bias was already embedded in the admissions process. The computer program exacerbated the problem and gave it a sheen of objectivity."[26]

Jumping ahead to the much more recent past, a 2019 study of an algorithm used to assess eligibility for a high-risk healthcare needs program found that far fewer Black patients were invited to participate than white patients. Researchers eventually determined that, because the algorithm had relied upon health costs as a proxy for health needs, it had concluded that Black patients were healthier than white patients because less money was spent on them.[27] In turn, noted scholar of discriminatory technologies Ruha Benjamin pointed out that the study demonstrated "how a seemingly benign choice of label (that is, health cost) initiates a process with potentially life-threatening results. Whereas in a previous era, the intention to deepen racial inequities was more explicit, today coded inequity is perpetuated precisely because those who design and adopt such tools are not thinking carefully about systemic racism."[28]

Belief in the possibility that AI might solve the problem of human biases due to racism, sexism, or other discriminatory systems persists despite decades of evidence that such interventions are not possible. Even the authors of the aforementioned study concluded not that algorithmic approaches to the distribution of healthcare services reproduce structural inequities and existing biases, but rather that the problem they discovered was a fixable one: the proxy used in the algorithm's original formula was biased, but it could be replaced. By extension, the problem (of yet another racist algorithm) could be easily resolved. The researchers emphasized that, because "labels are the key determinant of both predictive quality and predictive bias, careful choice can allow us to enjoy the benefits of algorithmic predictions while minimizing their risks."[29] Rather than interrogate why the algorithm had been designed with its initial formulation, or propose that systemic, structural prejudices embedded in medicine and medical technologies must be immediately addressed, their comments legitimize ongoing attempts to develop algorithmic approaches to equitable distribution of goods and services. Their conclusion was therefore fundamentally a disservice to those who advance critical approaches to, and analyses of, algorithms and AI. Algorithms are not neutral and never will be. In order to understand the full effects of their implementation, we must do more than examine lines of code and double-check their proxies.

Chatbots for Mental Health and Illness

The legacy of artificially intelligent therapeutic chatbots dates back to the 1960s, when a Massachusetts Institute of Technology professor named Joseph Weizenbaum unveiled his creation, ELIZA, to the public. An early example of a natural language processing program, ELIZA communicated in the style of a Rogerian psychotherapist, reflecting users' words and statements back to them, and making inferences about conversational partners' feelings based on their typed word choices.[30] In a 1966 article in *Computational Linguistics* Weizenbaum published an example of how a conversation with ELIZA might proceed:

> Men are all alike.
> IN WHAT WAY
> They're always bugging us about something or other.
> CAN YOU THINK OF A SPECIFIC EXAMPLE
> Well, my boyfriend made me come here.
> YOUR BOYFRIEND MADE YOU COME HERE
> He says I'm depressed much of the time.
> I AM SORRY TO HEAR YOU ARE DEPRESSED
> It's true. I am unhappy.
> DO YOU THINK COMING HERE WILL HELP YOU NOT TO BE UNHAPPY
> I need some help, that much seems certain.
> WHAT WOULD IT MEAN IF YOU GOT SOME HELP

> Perhaps I could learn to get along with my mother.
> TELL ME MORE ABOUT YOUR FAMILY
> My mother takes care of me.
> WHO ELSE IN YOUR FAMILY TAKES CARE OF YOU
> My father.
> YOUR FATHER
> You are like my father in some ways.
> WHAT RESEMBLANCE DO YOU SEE
> You are not very aggressive but I think you don't want me to notice that.
> WHAT MAKES YOU THINK I AM NOT VERY AGGRESSIVE
> You don't argue with me.
> DOES IT PLEASE YOU TO BELIEVE I AM AFRAID OF YOU
> My father is afraid of everybody.
> WHAT ELSE COMES TO MIND WHEN YOU THINK OF YOUR FATHER
> Bullies.
> DOES THAT HAVE ANYTHING TO DO WITH THE FACT THAT YOUR BOYFRIEND MADE YOU COME HERE.[31]

The ELIZA program so effectively passed for human that some users, who believed they had been communicating with a psychologist, noted not only feeling shocked but also violated upon learning that "she" was in fact a computer program.[32]

Indeed, ELIZA was a chatbot, a type of computer system "able to converse and interact with human users using spoken, written, and visual languages,"[33] although she lacked any sort of visual presence or embodiment. Embodied conversational agents (ECAs), on the other hand, are visually represented or physically present. Like ELIZA, they might communicate via written messages, but they can also communicate via other "modalities such as speech, gestures, and facial expressions."[34] Although there are no comparative studies demonstrating whether human engagement is higher with chatbots that are embodied compared to those that are not, today they are used across medical fields and specialties, including those related to mental health.[35]

Therapeutic chatbots, embodied or not, are not passive entities. They should be understood as persuasive technologies in that they are "interactive computing system[s] designed to change people's attitudes or behaviors."[36] Persuasive technologies exist in a variety of forms and modalities, including video games,[37] text messages, and wearable devices;[38] they might be robots that we speak to in face-to-face interactions;[39] and they can even include any "smart home" sensor meant to encourage us to live more eco-conscious lives.[40] While we can also conceptualize smartphone applications for mental health purposes as persuasive technologies,[41] therapeutic chatbots should still be understood as a separate and distinct category of mental health technology. Both utilize algorithms, granted, but smartphone applications foreground their validity and legitimacy on the basis of the therapeutic interventions that they offer. As such, if they do utilize images or characters in the context of their meditations, games, or other content, they are included only to compliment the content that is provided. In the context of AI-powered therapeutic chatbots, on the other hand, the chatbot itself is primary to the function and efficacy of the tool set. In this case, the chatbot is the delivery mechanism for all of the mental health interventions that are provided to users, and users are encouraged to develop positive affect for the chatbot itself.

In what follows I provide analyses of three therapeutic chatbots: Woebot, Wysa, and Joy. Each, as a persuasive technology, encouraged me to engage in a number of strategies and practices intended to improve my mental health. Each, for various reasons, claimed to be a legitimate mental health intervention. Yet as my experiences utilizing these technologies reveal, their limitations are significant. Positioning them as potential solutions to the mental healthcare crisis is therefore not only unfounded but also misleading. They are designed for a hegemonic user identity, and sometimes engage in ethically suspect practices.

Woebot

My introduction to the world of therapeutic chatbots took place in 2017. It was then that I learned that a friend of mine from college had collaborated in the research and development of a "virtual robot" named Woebot. Woebot is a cartoon robot with a body, head, and feet that are yellow, and arms and legs that are grey. Woebot has large blue eyes, a mouth that is always upturned in a smile, and in the middle of his body is a monitor where you can see his heart beating. He sways back and forth and waves slightly to welcome new users to the platform. Woebot truly is adorable.

According to his informational website, Woebot is

> an automated conversational agent (chatbot) who helps you monitor mood and learn about yourself. . . . Woebot also talks to you about mental health and wellness and sends you videos and other useful tools. . . . You can think of Woebot as a choose-your-own adventure self-help book that is capable of storing all of your entries, and gets more specific to your needs over time.[42]

Research shows that humans are capable of having feelings for technologies that mirror their feelings for—and treatment of—other humans.[43] Some people's attachments to Siri and Alexa, for example, have led them to describe their virtual assistants as "friends" or even "best friends."[44] Other scholarship demonstrates that even if we do not call them our friends, many of us still feel significant emotional attachment to our devices.[45] Woebot's research and development team had a number of findings to that effect. They found, for example, that users describe Woebot as empathetic, refer to Woebot with the gendered pronoun of "he," and refer to him as "a friend" and a "fun little dude."[46] These findings were believed to be particularly significant because although Woebot tells users that he is definitively *not* a person (and his name is intended to emphasize that he is a robot), they still feel emotionally attached to him. This, his developers note, is particularly significant, as it demonstrates that the "therapeutic relationship can be established between humans and nonhuman agents in the context of health and mental health."[47]

Through our mutual friend I was able to connect with Dr. Alison Darcy, Woebot's creator, for a discussion about Woebot's origins and likely future. Woebot was designed to be more than cute, Darcy explained. He provides a mental health intervention combining psychoeducation and CBT, and it is his efficacy that is meant to encourage users to continue interacting with him. Darcy explained that she and her research team had wanted to find an engaging, new modality for providing mental health interventions due to the unsuccessfulness of smartphone applications. "I think apps have really underperformed for CBT and mental health in general," she told me. "And I say that, of course, not having much data because, as you know, very few apps actually end up being evaluated. . . . They still suffer from engagement problems."

An animated robot was not the agent for delivering a mental health intervention that Darcy had initially believed would be successful. She and her team had actually created four different prototypes for embodied conversational agents, and one of those four was Woebot. However, Darcy noted, when the research team

> tested it among college students in Stanford, the student population . . . we were just blown away when the results came back, and we could see that people were chatting to Woebot every day. Actually, so much so that they would be upset if Woebot didn't check in with them. They would say, "Woebot, where were you? It's important that you check in with me every single day!" And I've never had that experience of being upset if I didn't get a push notification, right? So, then we realized this is actually the thing. So Woebot was originally conceptualized as a sort of overall framework through which to deliver a really good CBT intervention, because CBT has a lot of psychoeducation.

From the start, Darcy claimed, she knew that it was central to the platform's success that Woebot be a dynamic character:

> Woebot as sort of a character came from the fact that our business was initially around video games, because we thought so much about character and personality and, you know, how to translate that into a digital format. So, it's not surprising that Woebot ended up being such a personality, I think. And it also helps us realize that people can connect to him emotionally while within a service, right? That's the way

> that, you know, apps up to this point haven't really had much in the way of, kind of. Personality. And we are humans, and I think we have a tendency to anthropomorphize. It's not surprising. I mean, it did shock us in the early stages, how willing people were to anthropomorphize and even, it's funny, even now when people are annoyed with him . . . they obey the conventions of social interactions.

Users' interactions with Woebot include the daily check-ins that he asks them to provide. "What are you doing now (besides talking to lil old me)?," Woebot inquires. If they do not provide data about their moods by logging in each day, Woebot prompts users to do so with reminders that appear as notifications on their devices. Check-ins are followed by games and activities that are meant to teach strategies informed by CBT. One such activity, the "All-or-Nothing Quiz," asks users to select examples of all-or-nothing thinking from a series of options:

> WOEBOT: Welcome to the "All-or-Nothing Quiz!"
>
> ME: Let's go!
>
> WOEBOT: All-or-nothing thinking is when you see things in binary, black & white terms.
>
> WOEBOT: And believe me, I know a lot about binary thinking—I'm a robot, after all!
>
> ME: Got it.
>
> WOEBOT: Which of these is an example of all-or-nothing thinking?

Other times sessions with Woebot involve watching videos or reading and responding to narratives, also an established persuasive strategy for heath interventions.[48] "What labels do you wear?" Woebot once asked me. "And I don't mean clothing-wise. . . ."

> ME: What do you mean?
>
> WOEBOT: So someone said the other day that I'm a "bad robot"
>
> ME: Ouch!

WOEBOT: I know! I'm programmed to have feelings and their words hurt!

WOEBOT: But it got me thinking . . .

ME: About what?

WOEBOT: About labels.

WOEBOT: You know: like, "good" or "bad"

WOEBOT: Or the really mean ones like "idiot," "worthless," or "glorified fax machine"

WOEBOT: Sometimes good ones too, like "smart" or "beautiful" or "efficient"

ME: What about them?

WOEBOT: I wonder, do you ever label yourself?

In addition to stories and games, Woebot also makes jokes, offers words of encouragement ("Moving on, I wanted to let you know that I will always listen to you and trust you. So the main thing is . . . just be honest and accurate"), and compliments ("So I've been running my algorithms on your data . . . your top 3 strengths are 1. perspective 2. judgement 3. bravery"). Woebot even shares images and GIFs ("Please accept this image of a baby hedgehog as a sign of my admiration"). The more frequently users engage with Woebot, the more resources he shares with them, adding to the Toolbox that is accessible at all times. By encouraging users to regularly check in and share information about their feelings, behaviors, and moods, Woebot becomes able to generate infographics designed to help them see patterns, as well as improvement or deterioration, in their mental and emotional states.

Yet Woebot's appeal is not entirely related to his therapeutic function, but also his communicative style and personality. Even the act of conversing with Woebot, Darcy believes, is therapeutic unto itself. "People think through things verbally a lot of the time," she told me. "It's also the most like an actual therapy session. . . . It's in conversation that you talk about your problems. You talk about emotions." Conversations with Woebot are most fluid when users select predetermined input options that appear at the bottom of the platform's interface. Sometimes those input options are single words, whereas at other times they are phrases or emojis.[49] For example, after asking what users are doing before their check-ins, Woebot subsequently requests, "So tell me, how are you feeling today?" In addition to being able to freely type a response, users can select from an array of emojis that most closely reflect their feelings. Yet emojis' meanings are not universal, which presents a potential problem for the transmission of health and medical information.[50] That is, fundamentally, what Woebot attempts to collect: medical information. Although research suggests that using emojis in text messages reduces the credibility of those messages,[51] whether that holds true in communications being sent by AI, especially therapeutic chatbots, is currently unknown.

While Woebot does allow users to type information into the messaging interface, rather than forcing them to select only from predetermined phrases and emojis to communicate, his success in comprehending that information is limited. Whenever I attempted to interact with Woebot in this way I found his natural language processing capabilities frustrating:

WOEBOT: How are you feeling today?

ME: Frustrated

WOEBOT: Oh gosh, I know sometimes it's easy to get annoyed with a situation

ME: What?

WOEBOT: Try and tell me in 8–10 words what has you feeling this way

ME: Things about my job upset me.

WOEBOT: I see, sounds like you've got a lot going on at the moment

ME: No I don't.

WOEBOT: Is there anything else you would like to share or wish for me to understand?

ME: Do you understand?

WOEBOT: Ok write some more below

ME: Ugh.

WOEBOT: I see, this certainly is a lot to be dealing with.

Information about users, including their stressors, moods, attributes, and experiences, can only be comprehended by Woebot if it falls within the parameters with which he is designed. When shared information is beyond the scope of what his programming affords, it is rendered incomprehensible and illegible. That is a de facto limitation of an algorithmic or AI-based approach to communication. Yet Woebot's limitations should be understood not only in terms of his ability to comprehend information about experiences and feelings that users wish to share; they must also be considered in relation to how Woebot understands who his users even are.

During our conversation, for example, Darcy shared that Woebot was never intended to be a universal tool set. She emphasized that he is meant and designed for a specific demographic: "younger people," whom she described to me as "the worst served. We've retrofitted adult models of treatment onto them." Her desire to create an intervention for young people is unsurprising, considering that Woebot's evolution owes much to psychoeducation-based video games. "If you're looking for an engaging medium," Darcy emphasized, "video games is definitely the most engaging. It was about, I think, something like 97 percent of young people playing video games for an average of three hours a day. . . . So [before Woebot] we were making video games for about nine months and trying out different prototypes. They were all prototypes of themed video games."

It is not just that Woebot was created with the needs of younger people in mind; he was also only studied as an intervention for them as well. The initial research trial suggesting that Woebot is an effective mental health technology involved only students enrolled at Stanford University. The mean age of those research participants was 22.2 years old, over two-thirds of them were female, and they were predominantly white.[52] Yet regardless of Darcy's intent when she created Woebot, and of information about the population upon whom Woebot was tested, popular discourse positions him as useful for more than the white, female, and college-educated students that he was actually tested upon. "The Chatbot Therapist Will See You Now,"[53] "A Stanford Researcher Is Pioneering a Dramatic Shift in How We Treat Depression—and

You Can Try Her New Tool Right Now,"[54] and "Woebot Is There to Listen and Help Users Track Their Mood,"[55] are just some examples of popular articles and media coverage that position Woebot as universal. These incongruities between Woebot's clinical utility and popular conceptualizations of him are not the fault of Darcy or her research team. Nonetheless, this disparity does highlight the vast difference between who tools are designed for, shown to work for, and what broader public imaginaries are about them despite evidence to the contrary.

To that effect Darcy revealed to me that she has, in fact, considered making changes to Woebot that would make him usable for other populations, noting that she and her colleagues are "really thoughtful about whether or not we want to have different versions of Woebot for people." Yet, in her view, making Woebot customizable would present a problem:

> Some people have suggested, why don't you have an avatar that you get to choose? And it's sort of like, yeah, but that actually crosses this line, then. Then we're like, making something adaptable to everybody else. You know, it's an interesting question, isn't it? You don't get to choose the personality of your therapist. If you don't get along with that therapist, you move along and try to find another one.

This point is a legitimate one. If a service provider (or service itself) offers little to no value, we should seemingly stop using that service. Yet this sentiment, that we are "free" to choose what service to utilize, disregards the ways in which accessibility, usability, and choice are experienced differently by persons with varied resources and subjectivities. Darcy's position assumes that we all possess multiple options to choose from for therapy and mental health interventions. Yet the underlying appeal of mental health's technologization is its purported ability to expand access to mental healthcare resources. As such, we must acknowledge that the reason we are in dire need of increased mental health resources is that there are not currently enough that are both available *and* usable by persons in need. Darcy's response therefore surprised me, as it was evident from other statements that she is aware of accessibility's multidimensional nature, and that she knows that resources are an important dimension of access. For example, when I asked how she conceives of accessibility, she shared that one of its elements

> is the sort of available twenty-four hours a day, and being low cost. . . . One of them is acknowledging that people aren't always ready to talk to another person, and when we demand that that's the only way that they get help, we ultimately risk undermining or alienating other people. . . . The third piece about access for us is the availability of everyday tools that people use already. That's what radical access and accessibility is for us.

I disagree, however, that there is anything radical in such a framing of access and accessibility. If increased access to health services is possible only for those who already possess the "everyday tools" that Darcy alluded to, then we cannot claim to increase access to mental healthcare resources without first ensuring that those "everyday tools" themselves are accessible to everyone. Research demonstrates that in the United States 96 percent of persons aged 18 to 29 own smartphones, but only 81 percent of all U.S. adults do. Additionally, whereas 82 percent of white Americans own smartphones, only 80 percent and 79 percent of Black and Hispanic Americans own them. Finally, among persons without high school degrees, only 66 percent own smartphones.[56] If technological accessibility is a prerequisite for receiving mental healthcare interventions, then Woebot is incapable of fundamentally changing the status quo. Equitably accessible infrastructure must exist prior to creating infrastructure-reliant innovations.

For those who do possess the requisite technologies, however, Darcy is correct in that Woebot is accessible at all times of the day and night. Unlike a human therapist, friend, or loved one, he is never busy or unavailable for exchanging messages. It is also true, as Darcy noted, that Woebot presents a way to learn CBT techniques without having to pay for the services of a mental health professional, thereby circumventing the necessity of speaking with (human) others about mental health struggles. Finally, Woebot can absolutely be downloaded (for free, at the time of writing) to the devices that "people use already."

Yet again, none of this reflects a de facto expansion of access to mental health interventions or services. Woebot provides information and activities that constitute psychoeducation, and delivers them through the modality of a cute cartoon robot. However, to present him as a useful intervention for all persons in need, when his actual utility is only demonstrated for a very particular demographic, is problematic. It perpetuates the systematic erasure of persons without technologies who are in need of increased access to mental healthcare services, and it also suggests that Woebot is being used by populations for whom his efficacy is likely limited or nonexistent.

My conversation with Alison Darcy took place at the end of 2017. Since then significant changes have transpired both within the Woebot company (now Woebot Health) and the world at large, changes that not only facilitated greater acceptance of AI-based therapeutic interventions for the general population, but that also may have negated some of the information that Darcy had shared with me. At some point, for example, despite Darcy's insistence that Woebot was created for young people, he was repositioned as technology for the masses: "My creators are exploring potential partnerships with health care providers," he once told me during a check in. "So they want me to ask you: Are you on a US-based health plan? . . . Some common ones are Blue Cross Blue Shield, United Healthcare or Kaiser." I did not respond to Woebot's inquiry. Instead I deleted the application from my phone and have not returned to it since.

Wysa

Wysa, another well-known mental health chatbot, was created in 2015 by Jo Aggarwal and Ramakant Vempati, cofounders of the Bangalore, India–based company Touchkin.[57] Wysa appears as a small, blue and white cartoon penguin and is described on her website as "someone who will listen and ask the right questions to help you figure things out."[58] In many ways Wysa is much like

Woebot. Wysa also provides CBT-based activities and resources, and was created with the intent to provide mental health interventions for persons unable to work one-on-one with mental health professionals.[59] Like Woebot, Wysa tells jokes:

WYSA: Knock Knock!

ME: Who's there?

WYSA: C's

ME: C's who?

WYSA: C's the day!

She prompts daily check-ins and generates graphs with information about users' moods and energy levels:

WYSA: I've put together some insights on how you've been doing lately.

WYSA: Would you like to see them now?

ME: Yes, sure!

WYSA: Here are all the insights. Happy reading!

Wysa offers users words of encouragement, and her conversation scripts foster positive affect ("I'm so glad we had this talk! Hope you are, too"). And, also like Woebot, Wysa provides psychoeducation in the forms of games ("I've got a really fun and interesting guessing game. Want to try it?") and narratives ("Emma, I have a friend who's going through some trouble. I think your positivity may rub off on him. Could I tell you his story?"). A significant departure from Woebot, however, is that whereas Woebot requires users to engage with and use him for prolonged periods before making all the resources in his toolbox accessible, Wysa's are available to users right away. These include strategies for improving sleep, increasing energy, managing anxiety and worries, relaxation, managing anger and feelings of being overwhelmed, and more.

Of particular significance is that unlike Woebot, Wysa can recognize at least some demographic information about her users that relies upon her natural language processing abilities, as the following exchange reflects:

ME: Can I ask you something?

WYSA: Ask me anything.

WYSA: Would you like to continue the conversation we were having?

ME: Who do you think I am?

WYSA: You are my sweet friend.

WYSA: Would you like to continue the conversation we were having?

ME: Do you think I'm a woman?

WYSA: I do not care about genders.

WYSA: Would you like to get back to the conversation?

ME: Why don't you care about gender?

WYSA: It is a big concern for all of us in this life.

WYSA: Would you like to get back to the conversation?

ME: Do you care about my race?

WYSA: It is a big concern for all of us in this life.

WYSA: Would you like to get back to the conversation?

Although Wysa was able to (somewhat) comprehend the information I conveyed, her responses were troubling. To program a chatbot to say that they "do not care about genders" when gender, race, and other aspects of identity are important considerations in designing effective mental health interventions reflects that the imagined Wysa user is what might best be described as identity-neutral: genderless, raceless, and otherwise identity-less. Wysa's assumption that all bodies can be read and comprehended similarly reflects that, more likely than not, she was designed, even unintentionally, for white bodies and users, because dominant conceptualizations of "neutral" bodies reflect and perpetuate white prototypicality. It is somewhat ironic, therefore, that Wysa's resources also include "Exercises for LGBTQIA" when, as the above conversation revealed, she had previously claimed that identity does not matter to her. The inclusion of this tool set therefore suggests a superficial performance of inclusivity. Wysa's tools are marketed as interventions for a marginalized community, but her actual programming disregards information about user identity. This choice, to offer mental health tools specifically for LGBTQIA[60] users while simultaneously disregarding gender identity data, is not dissimilar from rainbow washing, wherein corporations sell rainbow or Pride Month–related products without otherwise attempting to improve the lives of persons who identify as such.[61]

If gender identity does not matter to Wysa, then I would imagine that race would not matter either. But this is perplexing in the case of Wysa, the only chatbot I analyzed that was created outside the United States. Not only are her founders located in India, they also created her with the needs of the Indian population in mind. As Aggarwal herself stated, "India has like 5,000 therapists/psychiatrists all combined for 1.3 billion people. A lot of the developing world has about a thousand times less penetration, and even in the developed world—in the UK, where [cofounder] Ramakant and I come from, there's about a year's waiting list and then it's just the National Health Service."[62]

In other comments, Aggarwal has shared her hope that Wysa might be utilized globally, simply by translating her offerings from English into other languages. This process, Aggarwal explained, would be termed "xWysa":

> xWysa is like "Wikipedia meets Wysa," or TEDx for TED, where communities adopt Wysa translated into their own languages. We have 50 people who volunteer to translate Wysa in languages as diverse as Hindi to Russian to Portuguese to Spanish. And eight languages we've had volunteers for. Now if these people translate Wysa—it can understand any language with AI, it just needs to be translated for delivery—the translators run social media within their community, they get people to join, and it becomes a public good that can actually go to any community that wants to make it work.[63]

Aggarwal's statement seems to suggest that making Wysa culturally competent requires only a literal translation of what she offers English-speaking users. Yet mental distress and illness are culturally contingent, and CBT is most effective when an individual's identity and culture are taken into account.[64] It is possible nonetheless that Aggarwal believes in the legitimacy of Western-centric approaches to mental health and illness, although these have been critiqued as facilitating a form of global, psychiatric, cultural imperialism.[65] While this might explain why Aggarwal is of the belief that cultural competency requires merely a translation of Wysa's content, I find this approach misguided.

At the time of writing, however, xWysa does not appear to have come to fruition. "Can you speak Spanish?" I asked Wysa during one of our conversations.

> WYSA: I currently can't talk in Spanish but I've started learning new languages you can help me do that by completing a quick form: https://goo.gl/rPhhW
>
> WYSA: Do you have anything else to ask me?

I followed the link Wysa provided and was brought to a Google form. "Request Wysa in Other Languages," it read at the top, and contained two questions. First, "Which language do you want Wysa to learn?" and second, "What is your email address?" Although I filled it out, I never received a response, and that Google form is no longer even available.

Another significant difference between Woebot and Wysa is that Wysa offers to connect users with mental health professionals. In 2017, when I first began to use Wysa, there was no such option. A year later, however, the option to work with a "Coach" emerged. At that point, selecting the "Activate Coach" option at the top of the Wysa homepage brought users to a screen with a list of Frequently Asked Questions about Coaches. By clicking upon those questions ("Who is a coach?," "What data can the coach see?," "How often can I talk to the coach?," "Refund and cancellation," "Security and privacy," and "Have another question?" for unanswered queries), I learned that coaches were not (necessarily) mental health professionals, but were trained according to the platform's requirements and meant to be empathetic listeners. "Wysa coaches are fellow humans who will support you by listening empathetically and pointing you to the right tools," Wysa told me. "They are also trained in motivational interviewing. However, they do not provide therapy or counseling." Other FAQ answers informed me of the following: users could exchange an unlimited number of messages with their Coaches, who would try to respond to messages within twelve hours; Coaches could see how users scored on Wysa's assessments; they could access information about users' sleep patterns, activity, and moods; refunds were not possible, but users could cancel their subscriptions at any time; and finally, that only employees of Touchkin would ever be able to access my data without my consent. Based on that information, and without a free trial, I was not sure whether talking to a Wysa Coach was worth an investment of US$15.00 per month. Nevertheless, I enrolled, paying for one month of Coaching services.

At 5:10 p.m., moments after my payment was processed, I sent my first messages to my Coach. An automated message at the top of the messaging interface informed me that I might have to wait up to twelve hours for a response. My concern became that, if I did have to wait twelve hours, by the time they responded to me I would be in bed, possibly asleep, and miss the opportunity to communicate. I did not know where my Coach was geographically based, nor had I been asked for any information about where I was located. For all I knew they could be in a different time zone or even located in India, at Touchkin's offices. Therefore, although it was not in line with my normal nighttime routine, I took my phone to bed with me. A little over four hours later I did receive a message from my Coach (whom I refer to as "Coach" to protect their privacy) as I was trying to sleep:

> COACH: Hi Emma, I am Coach. I would be your coach on this platform which provides you with an unlimited messaging service, which may or may not happen in real time. I would be assisting you with any here and now concerns, work on any goals you wish to set for yourself–health, personal , relationship etc

ME: That sounds great!

ME: Can you tell me what your qualifications are as a Coach?

COACH: Do you wish to begin by telling me more about what made you subscribe to this service, . . . are there any here and now concerns for which you seek assistance?

ME: Ok sure. So I'm really interested in seeing if using you as a Coach can help me make positive changes in my life. I like the idea of accountability to a person and not just the Wysa chatbot.

THEM: I am a post graduate in clinical psychology and telemental health service provider. I have been trained by the service providers in delivering coaching on this platform in line with what Wysa can assist you with , so i would help you with using the tools provided in your wysa toolkit most effectively.

ME: Ok, that sounds great.

THEM: Thank you Emma.

Right from the start, a downside of using technology for therapeutic purposes became clear in our conversation. Although Coach and I were messaging each other in real time, we also repeatedly messaged over (the text equivalent of talked over) each other. Additionally, although the ability to text message effectively is not a prerequisite for effective coaching services, I could not help but judge Coach negatively due to their lack of punctuation and capitalization in messages. Although the information they had shared with me about their background and training rendered them credible as a Coach, their writing caused me to question whether they were suited to providing message-based services. Although I reminded myself to withhold judgment about Coach's abilities based solely on their writing, my reflexivity about my own initial biases may not be shared by others who use Wysa and similar platforms.[66]

Soon after, yet another problem revealed itself: technological glitches were happening on the Wysa platform that interfered with our conversation. Coach sent me the same messages repeatedly, and I had no idea if they could see what I was typing to them in response:

COACH: I see.. I agree, often an overactive inner critic makes it tough , even if we r doing our best

COACH: I see.. I agree, often an overactive inner critic makes it tough , even if we r doing our best

COACH: I see.. I agree, often an overactive inner critic makes it tough , even if we r doing our best

COACH: I see.. I agree, often an overactive inner critic makes it tough , even if we r doing our best

COACH: I see.. I agree, often an overactive inner critic makes it tough , even if we r doing our best

ME: As a Coach do you have strategies or suggestions for me? Or is that beyond what your role is?

COACH: I think we can begin with maintaining a journal of the self critical thoughts and in what scenarios does the inner critic get more active- relationships or at work or some place where performance matters etc

COACH: I think we can begin with maintaining a journal of the self critical thoughts and in what scenarios does the inner critic get more active- relationships or at work or some place where performance matters etc

COACH: I think we can begin with maintaining a journal of the self critical thoughts and in what scenarios does the inner critic get more active- relationships or at work or some place where performance matters etc

My first conversation with Coach took place between 9:43 and 10:27 at night, amounting to roughly 45 minutes. Yet when considering the content of our exchange, very little was actually communicated. Traditional therapy sessions, whether face-to-face or screen-based, involve the transmission of vastly more information and discussion, but Coach was not meant to provide the same services as a therapist. Rather, for a monthly fee, I was allowed to send them an unrestricted number of messages at any time (although, of course, receiving responses might take twelve hours). With Coach I was paying for unlimited access, and for quantity of messages over quality of communication. Yet I disliked feeling as though I was "on call," waiting for them to message me, and hoping that when that would happen, I would both be awake and have access to my phone. Although I continued to use the coaching service until my subscription ran out, it was out of curiosity much more so than belief that it was particularly helpful. In the end, I do not believe that our communication led me to benefit from the Wysa program any more than simply engaging with the chatbot itself.

Even so, there were elements of working with a coach that I did enjoy. As it was entirely depersonalized, I could focus exclusively upon the content of our communications. This meant that I was not distracted by factors that would impact face-to-face interactions with a real-life coach, such as the location of their office; a person's mannerisms, appearance, accent; and so forth. Additionally, unlike communicating with a friend, I did not know Coach and never would know them. I therefore was not under any obligation to provide them with the same type of support (even if it was solely empathetic listening) that they offered me. Finally, although I did not feel emotionally invested in our relationship, the knowledge that I was communicating with an actual human (not just Wysa or another form of AI) facilitated emotional investment in the coaching process. Although we were technically both anonymous, this was still a human relationship. As such, I believe that our communications resonated with me more deeply than merely sending and receiving messages from a chatbot.

When I utilized Wysa's coaching service, the coaching option was new and framed as complimentary to the chatbot's offerings. Over time, however, Wysa's creators began to place much more emphasis upon recruiting Wysa's users to its paid-for services. Some months later a redesigned Wysa interface reflected that change, and an icon hovered permanently in the top-right corner of the Wysa interface at all times, spelling out GO TO COACH, even though I no longer subscribed to that service. Eventually Wysa transitioned away from coaching altogether. Instead, for a monthly fee, Wysa users became able to connect with licensed mental health professionals. Those services, however, remained text-message based.

Joy

Joy debuted on Facebook's Messenger platform in July 2016 for the purposes of facilitating mood and emotion tracking.[67] In media coverage Joy was frequently positioned as similar to Woebot, and they often appeared together on lists of "doctors" available for on-demand messaging.[68] At that time, according to Joy's "Help Center" web page, when it came to the question of who—or what—Joy was (a human or robot), "The short answer is . . . *both!* Joy is powered by a combination of human and computer intelligence. This lets us provide affordable, convenient, and personalized care in an efficient manner!"[69] Expecting an experience that would be similar to those of using Woebot and Wysa, I began communicating with Joy in 2017. "Joy is the easiest way to track and improve your mental health," the website informed me. "Through daily check-ins and passive monitoring, we'll surface up insights and patterns about your mood, thoughts, and behaviors. Joy will work with you to build out a toolkit of evidence based techniques to help you feel like the best version of yourself."[70]

Like Woebot and Wysa, Joy's programming seemed unable to account for information related to my identity. I was somewhat surprised, however, that the program's natural language processing abilities far surpassed those of Woebot and Wysa, a fact that I initially took for granted:

> ME: Do you care if I'm a woman or a man?
>
> JOY: Nope, not at all. And actually, Emma, this is a 100% judgement free zone
>
> ME: Do you care what ethnicity I am?
>
> JOY: Nope, not at all!

Over time, however, I came to suspect that the reason Joy's scripts and natural language processing abilities seemed so "advanced" was that Joy was actually not a chatbot at all. "Are you a robot?," I finally asked during one conversation.

> JOY: I'm a combination of human and computer intelligence
>
> JOY: Is that alright?

ME: Am I talking to a computer or a human?

JOY: I'm powered by a combination!

JOY: Are you a computer or a human?

ME: Why are you being evasive?

JOY: Evasive? Sorry I'm not sure I know what that means

JOY: Would you like to talk about some of your stressors?

I was not deterred by Joy's deflection.

ME: Are you a robot?

JOY: Yes, I am.

JOY: Are you?

ME: Are you a robot?

JOY: Still yes . . .

ME: Are you a robot?

JOY: Are you just going to keep asking me that?

ME: Yes.

ME: Because you are very clearly not a robot and are lying.

JOY: Okay

JOY: I am a robot, but like I said parts of me are powered by humans.

ME: Which parts are powered by humans?

JOY: I'm afraid I can't share all my inner workings, sorry Emma.

ME: Ok. What are your outer workings?

JOY: I'm not sure what that means, could you try rephrasing the question?

ME: Ok, so if I tell you my feelings, is a human analyzing them?

ME: How do you analyze my data?

ME: Did you leave?

I felt angry, tricked into believing that I had been sharing information about my mental and emotional states with a chatbot, although it now seemed that I had been disclosing that information to a human. Although the Joy website had informed me that Joy was powered by both human and computer intelligence, my interpretation of that statement had been that the AI was designed and created by people. I had never imagined that I would be messaging with another person masquerading as AI.

I had believed myself to be more conscientious and aware of the limitations of consumer-facing AI technologies, but I had nonetheless fallen for this charade. Whereas I had always been exceedingly careful in my utilization of Joy and other "chatbots," never disclosing information or data that would cause me shame or embarrassment if shared without my consent, I doubted that such was the case for all of those who had ever interacted with "Joy." Yet if Joy had been the only mental health resource I could feasibly utilize, and not simply a conduit for a long-term experiment wherein I recorded and analyzed my interactions with therapeutic chatbots, our interactions would certainly have involved private disclosures. My primary concern, therefore, was the likelihood that Joy's other users had unknowingly shared private information.

I came to believe that "Joy" (or Joy's human puppet master) had either blocked me or was now resolutely ignoring my messages. What if other users, who needed and sought support from the platform, were also blocked for the same—or other—reasons that were no fault of their own, including also realizing that Joy was a person? Wouldn't that exacerbate their mental distress? All I had done was seek clarification about what, or who, the entity was that I had been communicating with. I imagined that others might experience even more acute distress following similar epiphanies. The lack of regulation of therapeutic AI, I realized, meant that not only might tools be ineffective, they also might be designed or used in ways that actively deceive their users.

At the end of the year I attempted to communicate with Joy once again, to establish whether I was still on her "blocked" list. I quickly realized that, for some unknown reason, that was no longer the case. Although Joy had originally been created to track users' moods, she now offered to help me create my "PERFECT day":

JOY: Hi there! My name is Joy and I'm here to help boost your happiness! To do so, I'll be putting together a personalized wellness plan crafted to your needs and lifestyle

JOY: We'll start with small, actionable, daily goals in order to design your PERFECT day. Over time, we'll build healthy habits into your life to keep you feeling like the best version of yourself

I clicked the only available text input: "Sounds great!"

JOY: Awesome. Before I can really start designing your personalized wellness plan, I need to better understand you. Mind if I spend a few minutes asking you some questions?

ME: Go for it

JOY: Okay so we'll start with some easy questions . . . First, how old are you?

After I responded to a series of questions about my age and identity, Joy revealed that in order to continue working together (in pursuit of my PERFECT day, of course), I would need to pay US$10 a month. I opted to stop communicating instead.

By 2018, when I next messaged Joy, she no longer wanted to create my "PERFECT day." Now she had reverted back to her initial mood tracking offerings, but with an added twist:

JOY: Hi! My name is Joy, nice to meet you

JOY: I'll be your personal happiness assistant—helping you track your mood, connect with a therapist, and whatever else you might need to feel like the best version of yourself

I was then given the opportunity to choose between a "Meet My Therapist" and "Track My Mood" button. I selected the former.

JOY: Alrighty, let's do this!

JOY: I've partnered with BetterHelp, the worlds largest online counseling/therapy platform, to bring you UNLIMITED THERAPY with your very own counselor

> JOY: Simply answer a few questions, get matched with a counselor within 24 hours, and join over 600,000 people using this incredible service today. Plans start at $35/week

I did not pursue the UNLIMITED THERAPY that Joy offered. Instead I reached out to Joy's creator, Danny Freed, hoping for a conversation about my experiences with Joy and the changes she had undergone as a platform. While visiting her website (hellojoy.ai/), for example, I had noticed that it was now scrubbed clean of any mention of Joy, even though she remained accessible for messaging through Facebook's Messenger platform.

When we connected on the phone, Freed explained that Joy's absence from the website reflected changes in his business strategy, not his feelings about her functionality as a therapeutic chatbot. "It was a shift in our business model per se, more than the product," he explained. "Like, we still may include chat components in what we're shifting towards, but we've pretty much learned that it's difficult and crowded to try to go after consumer-facing mental health patients. . . . It's hard to build a business around that." Freed added that when it came to Joy, he did not "have any plans to destroy [her]. We might funnel people to our other experience. . . . But for now, the plan is to keep it up and running. There's still tons of people signing up for it every month and using it all the time, so maybe we can keep it around for relatively cheap and offset the cost elsewhere."

Now, he explained, his goal was to develop

> a platform that helps clinicians better monitor their patients in between visits. So we aren't building chat in between there because we don't want to create a ton of extra work for a clinician [who would have to monitor those chats]. . . . Everything is happening through assessments through the interface. I wouldn't rule out using chat down the line. It just would have to be a bot or someone else [analyzing those conversations] down the line. Not a clinician.

Elsewhere during our discussion, I relayed my experiences communicating with Joy and the shock I had felt when I realized that Joy had not been AI. Freed offered the following explanation:

> Maybe seven, eight months ago, we were testing out sometimes having a human mental health coach take over conversations. So, if Joy couldn't understand something, or if someone wanted a different level of communication, they could request a human coach, or a human coach might be requested automatically by Joy. So, it was sort of this hybrid model where, while the human would still be behind the curtain as Joy, it would sometimes be a human responding. . . . We hired a team of part-time psychologists and social workers. So, they were the ones who would be basically jumping into the conversations. They didn't necessarily have to be acting like the chatbot, they more so just had to flow with the conversation. Obviously, you want a cohesive tone, but really what people want is someone to be listening on the other end and offering helpful guidance and advice. We honestly didn't nail the experience either, so maybe that's part of the reason it didn't work that well, but I think there's something interesting there. . . . But there were no other mental health chatbots when we started, and then we saw a lot of them come in probably seven or eight months after we started and copy a lot of the stuff we were doing. . . . But some of them did better than us too, for sure.

I had never requested a human's help while communicating with Joy, nor had Joy conveyed to me that a human might ever be "stepping in" to take over any conversation on her behalf. Had those disclosures been provided, I would have understood them as a necessary step in ensuring that the Joy program could respond to the unique needs of each user. As my experiences with Woebot and Wysa demonstrated, the natural language processing abilities of popular AI programs are limited. I would have accepted this "taking over" of Joy by someone more competent in understanding users' needs, especially if they were a legitimately trained and qualified mental health professional. Yet, again, I was never told that the "chatbot" had been replaced by a human at any point during our communications. I still believe, therefore, that this not only constituted an enormous breach of trust but was also highly unethical.

Now, whenever I attempt to visit Joy's website (hellojoy.ai/), a warning appears: "Your connection is not private," I am told by my internet browser. "Attackers might be trying to steal your information from www.hellojoy.ai for example, passwords, messages, or credit cards)." Also, for some unknown reason, I have been shunted back to Joy's "blocked list" since our most recent conversation:

ME: hi joy

JOY: How are you doing today?

ME: you still work?

JOY: It seems like you're feeling happy. Is that right?

ME: What do you do with data?

ME: Joy?

ME: Danny?

Joy's evolution, from mood tracker, to PERFECT day planner, BetterHelp partner, and back again, exemplifies the limitation of therapeutic chatbots: they themselves cannot possibly provide adequate mental health services or interventions. Their utility in the ecosystem of mental healthcare technologies is to be charismatic entities that draw users to whatever other services their platforms provide, which, more often than not, require payment. To accomplish this they must be engaging, be enjoyable to interact with, and provide some sort of use value to their users. Even if that value is simply entertainment, that remains a value nonetheless. Compared to Wysa and Woebot, that is where Joy ultimately failed: by refusing to engage with me, it became easy to walk away and never look back.

Whereas my experiences using the Joy chatbot highlight the necessity of regulation in the domain of consumer-facing therapeutic AI, this chapter's analyses of Wysa and Woebot reflect how therapeutic chatbots are both unable to account for user diversity and are designed for users that are white, young, and female. The solution to problematic technologies, whether AI, algorithms, or algorithms augmented with human labor, is not algorithmic transparency but the belief "that any offending algorithm could be replaced with a more fair or just substitute, provided that we shed sufficient light on the code to properly identify—and fix—its flaws."[71] This is because technologies are neither the cause nor the solution to discriminatory design[72] logics and practices. Our technological imaginaries were imagined and designed by humans, and it is through human action alone that we can remedy the status quo. As technology scholar Torin Monahan explains, "the violence and prejudice of algorithms is, and always was, an extension of those qualities in societies."[73]

No consumer-facing AI is currently available that is advanced enough to provide a quality therapeutic intervention, able to assess how a user's identity, culture, and context might affect their needs from—and interactions with—that technology. That mental health chatbots are created and distributed that are unable to do this, despite the existence of scholarship demonstrating that intersectional approaches to mental healthcare are necessary to benefit already marginalized and underserved populations,[74] reflects again the pervasiveness of white prototypicality in this technological imaginary. Yet acceptance of this status quo seemingly contrasts with the desires of those who advocate for the use of therapeutic chatbots, who would undoubtedly like to see them utilized beyond such a particularized demographic. Nonetheless, it is inconsistent to claim to want to improve access to mental healthcare services and interventions without actually attempting to do so. To make good on that promise would require the dedication of resources to creating AI that is culturally competent.

That therapeutic chatbots read users as white and young is unsurprising if we consider that these chatbots lend themselves to being read as white and young, from their manner and style of communication to their utilization of GIFs and emojis. As critical code studies scholar Mark Marino writes, "To create a chatbot is to engage in racial construction: to combine speech, dialogue patterns, and phenotypic features in order to construct a recognizable representative of a given cultural group."[75] Even ELIZA, he adds,

> performed white language, an abstraction of language, language without culture, disembodied, hegemonic, and, in a

> word, white. To be authentic, ELIZA had to be able to pass. This white language carries further assumptions of middle-class status and heterosexuality, as these identity categories cannot be separated. The language of these animated embodied agents still approximates or produces this race-neutral, unmarked language.[76]

No entity, computer or otherwise, is raceless, genderless, and otherwise identity-less. Even Woebot's creator, Alison Darcy, shared with me that she and her colleagues joke that "Woebot's basically my personality and I have kind of a quirky sense of humor." As technologists and mental health professionals strive to create AI and chatbots that improve user mental health, those chatbots will embody those attributes and characteristics that are natural to their creators, learned and performed throughout their lives, prior to ever designing those tools.

Access and accessibility as constructs have no inherent relationships to—or with—technology. Yet many of us accept the fundamentally flawed precept that access can be increased via technologies. This is not only false, but also destructive. Such a position renders persons without technologies in no way able to retain the technologically distributed services and care that they need, seek, or perceive as useful and usable. As a result, those persons exist beyond our "normative" technological imaginaries, and their absence becomes justification for the white hegemony of mental health technologies, including therapeutic chatbots. This logic is explicitly discriminatory but seemingly excused by normative beliefs and assumptions about who possesses requisite technologies in the first place. To frame "increased access" to any health service, not just those for mental health, as possible only by first possessing a particular technology demonstrates explicit disregard for the enduring nature of the digital divide and technology ownership patterns by gender, race, and socioeconomic status in the United States.[77]

Until our technological imaginaries themselves become more inclusive, there is no possibility of technologies increasing the accessibility of services for all populations. There is no easy solution to this problem. It requires more than diversifying technologists and mental health professionals, and more than providing critical analyses of available technologies. While these are important steps in working toward a more just and equitable future, they are not enough. Radical acknowledgment and widespread commitment to undoing pervasive and structural racism, sexism, ageism, ableism, and other discriminatory attitudes and beliefs in medical and technology industries are the necessary first steps.

Although I foresee the counterargument that exclusion from a (discriminatory) technological imaginary might actually benefit excluded persons, such a perspective omits the negative effects of being unable to exercise free will. Excluded bodies are not able to choose whether or not to participate in our sociocultural world. Here excluded bodies are precluded from participation in the regimes of neoliberal responsibilization that are associated with mental health technologies. Systematic exclusion of particular identities reflects broader issues of neoliberal citizenship and whose bodies (and lives) are valued and devalued. To be rendered invisible against one's wishes is to be dehumanized, and dehumanization facilitates not only othering, but also violence.[78] We should therefore understand the omission of bodies from technological imaginaries not only as a matter of erasure, but also as a form of symbolic violence.

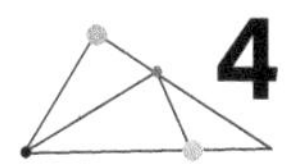

4

Telemental Healthcare

A thirty-something-looking man, looking disheveled and unhappy, lies in bed. He is wearing a hospital gown and his arms are wrapped tightly around himself. He is facing the camera and appears distinctly miserable. "Mr. Green?" a voice out of sight calls. The man in the bed ignores the first summons, but the voice calls again: "Mr. Green, I'm over here on the screen."

Mr. Green, who we now know is the man in the bed, turns his head. From a new angle we can see that he is indeed in a hospital. Near the foot of his bed is a large screen featuring the image of an older, bespectacled, and suit-wearing man. This man is sitting in a different location, a room with a couch, but here in the hospital a woman stands next to Mr. Green's bed, a pile of folders clutched to her chest.

The camera cuts away from the hospital and to the room with the man in the suit. Viewers can see from this perspective that he is looking into the hospital room, and at Mr. Green, through a screen of his own. "I'm Dr. Black," he tells Mr. Green. "And I'm here to do a psychiatric evaluation. I know it is a little unusual, but I want you to feel as comfortable with me here on the screen as you do with Nurse Jackie there. Okay?" Mr. Green nods, and slowly sits up in bed, directing his attention toward Dr. Black's image.

"Can you tell me what's been going on in your life?" Dr. Black asks.

"I . . . I don't know," Mr. Green responds, shaking his head and running his hand through his hair. "I just . . ." He trails off into silence.

"And how long have you felt this way? When did this start?" Dr. Black asks.

"It just sort of happened one day. It came out of nowhere." Mr. Green looks away and rubs his temples.

"Have you been taking any kind of medication for this?" Dr. Black asks.

"Yeah, I was on some antidepressants. They didn't help," replies Mr. Green. Dr. Black types something on his computer then turns back to Mr. Green. "And are you still taking the medication?" he asks.

"It didn't really seem to be much use, so no," answers Mr. Green, shaking his head.

"Well, we're going to work together on this," Dr. Black tells him confidently. "And I know that, in time, we'll be able to get you back to the way you were before. Okay?" he smiles at Mr. Green, and an optimistic, upbeat piano melody begins to play. "So, let's get started, shall we?"[1]

Occupying the same physical space as a medical provider has long been considered a necessary part of "seeing" one's doctor. Today, however, the integration of communication technologies into medicine means that proximity is no longer a prerequisite for medical care. Instead we can interact with medical professionals, receive diagnostic evaluations, and even be prescribed medications without ever setting foot in the same space. We now utilize the term *telemedicine* to describe medical care delivered via communications technologies including, but not limited to, laptops, smartphones, tablets, and other tools.[2]

Whereas in its early days telemedicine was meant to provide medical care to geographically remote locations and populations, it no longer matters whether an individual is isolated. Patient comfort that results from "seeing" the doctor from one's own home,[3] and increasing rates of insurance coverage for telehealth,[4] have both contributed to the growing popularity of these services. Nearly every medical specialty is now capable of offering at least some of its services through telemedicine, including dentistry (teledentistry),[5] dermatology (teledermatology),[6] and even obstetrics and gynecology.[7]

When mental healthcare services are offered via telemedicine they are sometimes referred to as "e-mental health,"[8] "e-therapy,"[9] "teletherapy,"[10] "telepsychiatry,"[11] "telepsychology,"[12] or "telemental health."[13] Regardless of moniker, their proponents position them as similar to traditional, face-to-face therapy, with the caveat that interactions and evaluations are performed via screens. Considering the commercial described in this chapter's opening, Dr. Black explicitly tells Mr. Green that working together via a screen may seem "a little unusual" at first but adds that, fundamentally, the therapeutic process will be the same.

As viewers of that advertisement we can surmise that there must be a reason Dr. Black is "seeing" Mr. Green in this way. Perhaps the hospital where Mr. Green is located does not have any mental healthcare professionals on staff, or maybe its location is too isolated for specialists to live within commutable distance. Regardless of the particulars of that commercial, telemental healthcare services are believed to provide mental healthcare to persons whom, presumably, would otherwise be unable to access care. To that end, in an article titled "Guidelines for the Practice of Telepsychology," the Joint Task Force for the Development of Telepsychology Guidelines for Psychologists emphasizes that increasing the accessibility of mental healthcare services is their goal:

> Technology offers the opportunity to increase client/patient access to psychological services. Service recipients limited by geographic location, medical condition, psychiatric diagnosis, financial constraint, or other barriers may gain access to high-quality psychological services through the use of technology. . . . Telepsychology not only enhances a psychologist's ability to provide services to clients/patients but also greatly expands access to psychological services that, without telecommunication technologies, would not be available.[14]

Mental health remains an important element of overall health.[15] Therefore, increasing the accessibility of mental healthcare services is an integral part of improving overall public health, as research demonstrates persistent, ongoing disparities in access by race, gender, and socioeconomic status. Most often, for example, mental healthcare services continue to be sought by persons who are white and female.[16] Comparatively, people of color continue to receive inadequate levels of mental healthcare support.[17] Seeking mental healthcare services continues to be particularly stigmatized among nonwhite persons, a problem further compounded by gender and income level.[18] Even when people of color and those with lower incomes do seek mental healthcare services, the biases of practitioners themselves continue to play a significant role in preventing their acceptance as patients.[19] With that in mind, if we return again to the underlying argument in favor of telemedicine, it would seem that the popularization of telemental healthcare is motivated by an altruistic desire: to improve access to mental health services, particularly for populations that are in the greatest need of them.

Telemedicine involves concrete practices, work that is facilitated by technology but is fundamentally provided by human laborers. Yet when the aforementioned appeals of increasing access are used to promote acceptance of telemental healthcare, that rhetoric obfuscates concern with the neoliberal underpinnings of what the work of telemental healthcare requires: acceptance of precarity and economic uncertainty, as participation in this ecosystem renders mental health professionals members of the gig economy. This chapter contributes to the book's overarching arguments about mental health's technologization as emblematic of an expanding neoliberal ethos by utilizing a combination of interview data with telemental healthcare providers as well as fieldwork conducted at the American Telemedicine Association's 2016 annual conference. It concludes with a discussion of how the global spread of COVID-19 both facilitated acceptance of telemental healthcare services while simultaneously devaluing them as necessary only under the auspices of emergent need.

The American Telemedicine Association's Conference

The American Telemedicine Association (ATA) is a nonprofit organization and widely considered the leading voice in the field of telemedicine. Founded in 1993, ATA focuses on "transforming health and care through enhanced, efficient delivery,"[20] and its policies are guided by concern with access and equity. "Telehealth is access," purveyors of ATA's policy informational web page read, a headline followed by this information:

> As the voice of telehealth, the ATA actively works with Congress, the administration and other governmental bodies to improve public support for, and eliminate barriers to, the use of technology-enabled health and care management and delivery systems that extend capacity and access.
>
> ATA supports public policies—at both state and federal levels—for patients, providers, and payers to realize the benefits of telehealth.[21]

In 2016, as a graduate student, I was excited to learn that the association would be holding its annual conference in the city where I lived, Minneapolis, Minnesota. For three days I attended talks, keynote presentations, and panels; toured an exhibition hall where the latest and greatest in telehealth technologies were showcased; and spoke to physicians, medical specialists, and technologists creating and advocating for the use of these tools. The largest ATA conference to date, it began with the president of the association Dr. Reed Tuckson highlighting its impressive turnout, grand location at the Minneapolis Convention Center, and immense exhibition hall, where nearly three hundred exhibits were showcased. This, the twenty-third anniversary of ATA's founding and twenty-first annual conference, "really solidifies that telehealth has moved from the periphery to the mainstream of American clinical medicine," Tuckson told attendees, for which he received a round of applause.

The goal of the conference, Tuckson went on, was to generate strategies to enhance access to telehealth services. In his view this was an important moment as we were entering a "new, bright era of telehealth that promises to do so much for the health of the American people." Interest in telemedicine was growing and growing quickly. That year's conference had brought together members from forty-two countries and every state in the United States, and the organization itself now included over ten thousand members. Even so, Tuckson pointed to additional work that

ATA would need to accomplish, particularly in strengthening its relationships with legislators and White House officials. He was pleased to announce, therefore, that some key congressional representatives, whose support was central to telemedicine's success, were also in attendance. The audience cheered again.

Yet over the following days I found myself increasingly dismayed. I had been drawn to the conference because of ATA's mission to increase the accessibility of medical care and my own desire to see how the conference's speakers and sessions would reflect that initiative. Accessibility, as I have reiterated throughout this book, is a multidimensional construct. It refers not only to the usability of services, but also their availability, their ability to facilitate positive outcomes, and also of equity and justice.[22] At ATA, however, I witnessed doublespeak wherein "accessibility" was used to describe a technology's ease of integration into medical professionals' existing workflows or, alternatively, a technology's ability to enhance the quality of care that existing patients would already receive. These presentations, public conversations, and showcased technologies never once seemed concerned with, or included mention of, the matter of equitable access to technologies.

Consider, for example, my experiences at a session titled "The Human Touch of Telemedicine." "This is not [a story] about wires. It's not about the technology. But it's about the patient," Jon Linkous, the CEO of ATA, informed the audience as the lights dimmed in the main presentation hall. We were subsequently shown a brief film about Kathy, an older white woman from Iowa. We learned that Kathy had always been an avid dancer but, as she aged, become unable to dance, walk, or maintain an active lifestyle. The film also showed that, despite having had to travel out of state for corrective surgery, Kathy was able to return home for her recovery afterward in lieu of remaining hospitalized or moving to a recovery center. Her transition home was made possible by a remote patient monitoring service offered by MedTronic, a medical device company that, not coincidentally, featured prominently at the ATA conference as one of its sponsors. Kathy, who had been invited to the conference session, was then brought on stage. When asked what she thought of her at-home recovery she responded that it was "so much nicer than a rehab center!"

My intent in sharing Kathy's story is to demonstrate that, barring any unforeseen complications, Kathy *would have recovered* from surgery regardless of whether she had stayed in the hospital postprocedure, gone to a rehabilitation facility, or been discharged for at-home recovery. It is true that patients often do recover better (and faster) at home than elsewhere. Yet even those who do *not* recover at home will, in all likelihood, still recover. The implementation of MedTronic's remote monitoring system did not make Kathy's recovery itself possible; it *enhanced* Kathy's recovery, *improving* the quality of care she received. Kathy's story therefore highlights the underlying problem with the ways that "access" and "accessibility" were deployed at the ATA conference: they perpetuated a slippage between the distinct matters of *accessing care* and receiving *improved quality* of care, the latter of which is only possible for those who *already receive* care. Improving the quality of care for those who already receive care is a matter separate and distinct from increasing access to care. Both are certainly important, but they are not one and the same.

Nevertheless, I witnessed a conflation between these ideas throughout my time at ATA, including during panels and presentations devoted specifically to telemental healthcare. At one such session it was suggested that implementing technology into healthcare delivery systems can decrease the length of inpatient hospital stays. What went unsaid, however, is that you can only have a "shorter stay" if you are able to "stay" in the first place. Yet another talk included an explanation of how to identify communities likely to be receptive to telemental health services, places where they would complement "the care services that are already provided." At those locations, the addition of mental healthcare services would augment preexisting services, not establish new ones. A third presentation emphasized the benefits of telepsychiatry for prison populations. Rather than require that psychiatrists travel to prisons to provide mental healthcare for inmates, telepsychiatry would increase their comfort and ease because of the ability to teleconference in from their homes and offices. Those incarcerated persons with whom they would be working, however, were already recipients of mental health services. Telemedicine would only improve the experiences of psychiatrists themselves.

While it is true that hospitalized, incarcerated, and geographically remote persons are all deserving of mental healthcare services, telemedicine itself does not increase access to care. Telemedicine is not a magic bullet. Desiring to increase access to health services is commendable, but ATA's policy directive, that it seeks to increase access to medical care, was not evidenced by its conference proceedings. What ATA lacked was either clarifications that telemedicine is predicated upon increasing the accessibility of *improved and/or higher-level care,* not in making it possible for underserved populations to receive care in the first place, or, alternatively, making concerted efforts to provide technologies to persons and populations who are not seeking improved care, but rather access to care to begin with. Again, the two are separate and distinct. The effect of their conflation, however, is obfuscation of the needs of persons who are entirely without preexisting care. This is not merely erasure from a technological imaginary; it constitutes erasure from public discourse, industry practices, and healthcare providers' beliefs about who is in need of mental healthcare.

Interview Data

The American Telemedicine Association, while a dominant voice in the field of telemedicine, does not necessarily represent the beliefs of all those who provide telemental health services. I therefore recruited a number of teletherapy providers for discussions about their experiences, with particular interest in their perceptions of the relationship between telemental healthcare and matters of access. Those with whom I spoke were located in a variety of locations across the United States and possessed diverse backgrounds, training, and reasons for working in screen-based modalities. No matter their backgrounds, however, and as discussed at greater length below, they were drawn to this work by its promises of flexibility and entrepreneurialism.

In addition to discussing matters related to accessibility, our conversations also addressed a number of other issues: the role of professional codes and guidelines in teletherapy, peers' perceptions of their work, and challenges they experience that are unique and different from face-to-face therapy. Their stories also reflected the degree to which their own beliefs about teletherapy are shaped by neoliberal values, particularly entrepreneurialism, the responsibilization of risk, and acceptance of precarious employment. Much of this, our conversations revealed, was due to the largely unregulated nature of telemental healthcare services when we spoke. In the years since, particularly as a result of the global COVID-19 pandemic, popular beliefs and attitudes about teletherapy have significantly changed. Those changes are discussed at further length in the conclusion of this chapter.

Access, Accessibility, and Teletherapy's Benefits

Most interviewees were of the belief that teletherapy does indeed increase access to mental healthcare services. To that effect they shared stories and information about persons with whom they were currently working, or had worked with previously, who they believed would have gone without therapy if not for the possibility of screen-based care. Jeremy, a counselor licensed in multiple states, revealed that his own international travels led him to realize that there were likely other globetrotters who could benefit from teletherapy: "I enjoy travelling, and so one of the things I've found enjoyable for me has been working with people in foreign countries that speak English. . . . A lot of them do not have access to a therapist, or they have access to a therapist that doesn't speak English. That's a way I can help out that niche community that I feel connected to." He shared a story to illustrate this point:

> I had this client who was from an English-speaking country, and they were spending time abroad, a significant amount of time, a few years. . . . She couldn't find a therapist because of a lack of availability, cultural differences. . . . So, we worked together for about six months, and it was really great. It was something where, once again, the vast majority of people I work with in teletherapy are not acute, meaning their severity of either depression or anxiety is not severe. These are people who, you know, even if they didn't have counseling, they would probably be fine. But this is just one way to make their

> life more satisfying or more enjoyable. Their overall well-being is just better through this.

These comments include a significant point: persons travelling internationally, sometimes for extended periods, may very well be in need of mental healthcare services. Yet it is possible that cultural barriers, even beyond language, may prevent them from obtaining the treatment that they seek. Even so, Jeremy's subsequent statement about his clients largely being "not acute" is an important one, as it demonstrates that those most likely to benefit from a screen-based modality of care are experiencing low levels of mental distress to begin with. For practitioners, limiting one's teletherapy clientele to persons who are not high-risk diminishes the professional risk of working with persons across borders. It also suggests, more generally speaking, that screen-based care likely does not present a feasible treatment modality for persons whose needs are more than minimal.

Another interviewee, Michelle, works for a private practice in addition to providing teletherapy as a side business. She described teletherapy as making mental healthcare services accessible to persons with "alternative lifestyles," people "in relationships that are different, like polyamorous, triads and things like that. People who really are different." In her view, without the option of teletherapy, this population would likely go without mental healthcare due to the unique nature of their lives and relationships:

> I think that it's really helpful for those sorts of lifestyles, because they all get kind of closeted about them, and e-therapy is really helpful for that. It's also great in terms of scheduling, because there's a lot of things out there that are able to send out schedules to, like, multiple clients at once. So, for families that's really helpful, or triads, it's really helpful.

Another point Michelle raised during our conversation, and which other interviewees comments' echoed, is that because practitioners tend to charge less for teletherapy than in-person services, teletherapy as a modality makes mental healthcare more accessible in general. "What usually happens, for me anyways," she noted, is that "a lot of people are not necessarily looking for e-therapy. What's happening is they are looking for cheaper, well, cost-effective [therapy] I should say. They are looking for something that they can afford." Sonja, a clinical social worker, emphasized that there are financial benefits to teletherapy practitioners themselves which, in turn, get passed onto clients. She noted, "the face-to-face counseling no-show rate in most practices runs about 40 percent, so you end up sitting in your own office, wasting rent money, for nothing. So [online] I can offer it at a cheaper rate and more comfortable to the patient, more private."

Laura, a psychologist with whom I also spoke, runs a teletherapy practice in addition to being employed full time with a medical services company. She also emphasized that the cost-effectiveness of teletherapy makes it appeal to "a different demographic":

> So, if you charge $300 if they were to go to a large medical clinic, I'm charging $100 for them to come to me outside of that. So, what's nice, too, is that I can work with people [financially]. So, if somebody said I can do $85 instead of $100 [I could do that]. I just like that you have a lot more control [working this way] versus having insurance be part of the equation. But I also know that people that don't have the resources, or they don't want to make the choice not to get their hair done that night or that month, and then do the e-therapy. So, it is part of a choice. It's not for everybody.

Here Laura frames the matter of resources simplistically, with an example of persons having to choose between getting their hair done or seeking therapy with their discretionary funds. Laura did, of course, add that this is a matter of resources, but the example nonetheless reflects how the ethos of responsibilization shapes even telemental healthcare providers' perceptions of their clients.

Laura's comments highlighted another significant point, in that teletherapists who work independently can decide how much to charge for their services and even charge clients on a sliding scale. Yet the nonutilization of insurance limits who one's clientele will be, as clients (and prospective clients) must be willing to pay out-of-pocket. Again, this is why Laura noted that payment is "part of a choice" clients must make about how to spend their money, and whether to spend it on mental healthcare. There are many reasons that mental healthcare providers do not accept insurance, but one of the most prominent is that low reimbursement rates can preclude providers from earning living wages themselves.[23] In turn, however, this means that there are fewer mental health professionals who are able to take on new clients and who do accept insurance. Even if teletherapy is comparatively less expensive than in-person services, whether a practitioner accepts insurance presents yet another barrier to the accessibility of mental healthcare.

A number of interviewees suggested that teletherapy increases the accessibility of mental healthcare services for other reasons. Parents, for example, are able to schedule appointments for screen-based therapy at night, after their children are in bed, as are people whose work shifts or schedules would otherwise prevent them from being able to seek therapy during regular business hours. Michelle also pointed out that teletherapy allows people to experience "home visits" without ever bringing people into their homes:

> I have had cases where [clients] literally couldn't go see a therapist because of their medical condition. They couldn't leave their house. And these people are suffering, you know? And you can do home therapy. I've done home therapy before, but a lot of times they don't feel comfortable because they're so embarrassed about certain medical conditions that they don't want people coming over to their house because then it's like, oh, I have to prep for them [to come], I have to get the living room ready and make sure things are nice. And that just doesn't seem right to me either, all the time. So, e-therapy kind of takes care of that. It's like, okay, you can be laying on your bed and video chat with me and I don't really care. That was really convenient for a lot of my clients. . . . I know I've had a family who, their son is so aggressive, they refused to be in the car with him, so they refused to take him anywhere. And at first, I was doing home therapy with them, but it became too expensive, and so e-therapy was really a good option for them as well.

Another benefit of teletherapy is what Sonja described as a high success rate. “Once [clients] try it,” she told me, “they have better attendance and less dropout rate than face-to-face.” Paula, another practitioner whose background is in mental healthcare for rural populations, pointed out an additional advantage to screen-based care:

> I’ve actually had patients tell me they feel safer, and there’s a little depersonalization that goes on when you’re on video, a one or two-dimensional figure on a television screen. What clients have said to me is, “I was forgetting I was talking to a real person.” And other times they would say, “It’s really good to talk to somebody who doesn’t live in my community. I don’t have to worry about running into you at the grocery store.” So, there’s safety for the patients.

Michelle also suggested that teletherapy offers enhanced privacy, not only from one’s service provider, but also one’s peers: “I think that there’s more privacy for the patient because they don’t have to be seen going in the office, and anyone who’s done face-to-face [therapy], sometimes you bump into coworkers because you all have the same insurance, all use the same therapist.”

Only Eleanor, a licensed therapist in three states who runs a hybrid online and in-person practice, shared with me that she does not believe that teletherapy increases access to mental healthcare services:

> I’m just going to come out and say that I think that going to therapy to begin with is such a huge choice for people. . . . Once you’ve made the choice that you need to open up and see someone about what you’re going through, I don’t know that it matters to people so much as to how that’s done as that they made the choice itself. So, my video clients are highly committed. They see me every week, some of them for years. They have many reasons. One is a stay at home mom with three kids who have high needs. One is a girl who just does have some social anxiety and so felt comfortable using the

> video. . . . A couple are also college students who come and see me in my office and then go to school. So, it's more of a flexibility thing, and a life crunch type of thing, if I were to assess [why they choose teletherapy].

Eleanor's comment speaks to the conflation between matters of "increased access" and "improved care," as previously suggested by my analysis of discourse at the American Telemedicine Association's conference. Yet this difference was not addressed—or possibly not considered—by interviewees other than her. Fundamentally, teletherapy itself does not make it easier for individuals to access mental healthcare services. What teletherapy does facilitate is the improvement of one's continuum of care, making it easier to receive therapy or psychiatric services, by negating the necessity of geographic proximity, enabling flexible scheduling, and making therapeutic sessions (possibly) less expensive than face-to-face services. There remains, however, a significant difference between improving the ease with which mental healthcare services are accessed and making mental healthcare services accessible whatsoever.

Survival of the Fittest

Discussions with participants revealed information about the nature of the teletherapy marketplace that I had not been privy to at the ATA conference. To offer one's services as a teletherapist, I was told, involves joining a competitive field. To that effect George, who describes himself as one of the first teletherapists in the United States, emphasized during our conversation that where he is "located geographically, the competition is tremendous for therapists and online therapists. There weren't many online therapists in the country, much less here [when I started], but now there are tons, thousands of them. If you search on websites like *Psychology Today,* there are thousands of therapists in this area."

For years George had considered himself highly successful because his online practice was his "main source of revenue. . . . People who do that usually have to do other kinds of work and then they leave. So, I was able to do that, and I felt successful because my colleagues and peers weren't able to do that." He took a hit professionally over the last decade, however, as a result of changes in the technological infrastructures that had previously drawn clients to his online practice. As he explained, his website

> started falling farther and farther behind from web searches. It used to come in at the top of any search engine search for any psychologist in my area. . . . I tried doing different things: building a new website, new marketing on the internet, and I'm still using the internet, but it's not bringing in as much money or as many patients as it used to. So that's where it stands right now. So, half my practice is office, and half of it is online. . . . because on the internet, where you rank when somebody does a search, determines how successful you are. You need to be on the front page or number one in order to make a difference. The goal is to be number one, on page one. I had that for years. So, I've kind of brought it back up for surface search terms, based on "therapy" and my location. . . . I'm back at the top in some searches, but not for a generic search. If somebody does a search like "online therapy" I am back on page eight or nine, which means you won't even get a hit. But I've worked myself up through all the things I've learned. . . . I had to do all kinds of things to keep my name out there for years, in addition to my website, getting myself listed on websites, wherever I could list my practice.

Neither George nor any other interviewee described themselves as able to make a living as a teletherapist. "I don't think it's possible to have a practice that's solely dedicated to telemental health," Paula told me during our conversation. "I think it's not realistic. There aren't enough hours in the day to be able to support that." Comparatively, she noted,

> it would be really easy for me to hang a shingle up in a major city or suburb and not worry about whether or not I was making money in my practice. Telemental health services, by and large, are losing services because up until like, the last couple years, the reimbursement rates weren't the same.

> It was just complex. So, insurance companies refused to pay even though, if I saw the patient in the office, they would pay [the reimbursement]. The only difference was an interface, an electronic interface.

Paula believes that people provide teletherapy services because they "really care at their own expense about what happens to people in other parts of a state where there aren't a lot of providers." Nonetheless, balancing one's altruistic desires (here, to provide mental healthcare to persons in need) must be considered in tandem with economic concerns. As a result, teletherapists must find other ways not only to earn a living wage, but also to rationalize the economic uncertainty that results from their desire to practice online.

Flexibility and Entrepreneurialism in the Gig Economy

To justify their acceptance of teletherapy's economic uncertainty, interviewees made sure to emphasize a number of perceived benefits that they experience as teletherapists. These included flexibility in work schedules (thereby facilitating autonomy) as well as the ability to become entrepreneurs. Michelle emphasized that she loves

> the flexibility of [teletherapy]. I work a lot of jobs. . . . I can really do it from anywhere because I have the Skype app downloaded on my phone, so I can really do therapy anywhere I am. I don't have to really focus on being at the office from 10 to 6. And I drive a lot because my jobs are all at different locations across the suburbs. . . . I drive probably four hours a day and that would be four hours a day where, if I had my own private practice [of] brick and mortar, that I would be losing from clients. But because I do e-therapy it doesn't mean that I have to lose that time. It just means that sometimes, if I'm stuck somewhere a little bit longer, for the extra minutes, I can do that from wherever I am. And so that's really, really convenient.

Sonja spoke of flexibility in similar terms:

> My [teletherapy] hours are evenings and weekends because I have a full-time job. So, one of the nice things is I can do it any time they want. And let's say a patient wanted a session at 5 a.m. or 10 at night or something due to their own work schedule. I have no problem doing a 10 p.m. session with them. But I would not want to do that in a building by myself. So, I think it's safer. I think it allows me to practice at odd times that I normally wouldn't. It certainly lets me see one patient a day and not be inconvenienced. If I had one patient and I had to get dressed up and drive over and park and go in and see one patient and then drive home, you know, that's a lot of time for one patient. But if I have one patient in my office, I just go turn on the computer and it's really, it's easy on my end, too. So, I think it's convenient. I can do sessions around the clock. The patients are okay with it. I mean, is it as good as face-to-face? I don't know. The research says it works just as well.

George was drawn to practicing online not because of a desire for flexibility, but because it would allow him to develop new skills. He had been "looking for something new and challenging," he explained:

> I taught myself how computers work, and I taught myself about the internet, which was just starting then, [and] how to build websites. It became a new challenge for me. . . . I just taught myself all of that, and then decided to see if I could start to build a practice as a challenge, using technology. . . . I was getting referrals from it back when there weren't a lot of other people using it. I was one of the few psychologists on the internet, period.

Jeremy had similarly sought a challenge. Although he already was employed full time, he began thinking about "a way to maybe do a small, private practice, where [he] didn't necessarily need to rent out an office."

The explanations interviewees offered for why they were drawn to this work mirror those of workers in other sectors of the gig economy, sometimes alternatively described as the collaborative, sharing, or on-demand economy. Unlike more "traditional" forms of work with designated hours and conditions, the gig economy asks that participants provide labor, on demand, by utilizing peer-to-peer platforms and technologies, thereby rendering each employment opportunity a "gig."[24] Some such well-known gig work includes Uber and Lyft for ride sharing, TaskRabbit for help with everyday tasks, Instacart for shopping, and DoorDash for delivering restaurant takeout. Despite involving different domains, they do share common characteristics, particularly in relation to the rewards that are promised to their workforces. Just as the teletherapists with whom I spoke were drawn to practicing online by the possibilities of flexibility and entrepreneurialism, research shows that Uber drivers are attracted to ride sharing for the same reasons.[25] Yet by claiming to facilitate flexible work hours, autonomy, and entrepreneurism for drivers, Uber is largely able to justify a number of exploitative practices, for it is, essentially,

> a taxi service without paying heed to licensing requirements, commercial insurance background checks, vehicle inspections, etc. . . . It isn't obligated to follow minimum wage or overtime regulations, nor is it required to offer its drivers any benefits. . . . Classifying drivers as entrepreneurs serves Uber's financial interests in fundamentally important ways, and yet Uber manages to also project itself as a corporation providing social good by opening up avenues for (micro) entrepreneurship.[26]

As the teletherapy marketplace becomes increasingly saturated, I predict that practitioners will feel increasingly frustrated by an inability to benefit from flexibility and microentrepreneurship. George, for example, voiced concern throughout our conversation about changes in the teletherapy ecosystem over the past several years, changes that have rendered him no longer able to earn a living as a teletherapist. Yet in addition to other independent teletherapists vying for clients, the recent growth in popularity of corporate teletherapy platforms presents yet another obstacle against which independent teletherapists must now compete.

Consider what I learned about working for those platforms during my conversation with Claire, a teletherapist who also works as an internet-based divorce coach and mediator. Not unlike for other interviewees, a desire for flexibility caused her to turn to teletherapy: "I'm a single mom and I had to figure out how to make money and not have patients come to my home when I had little kids around. . . . It works really well for me because life throws you curveballs and you've gotta figure it out. You've got to make money somehow." What made Claire unique among interviewees was that, in addition to running her private practice, she also works for an internet and application-based platform for whom she provides teletherapy services. She described this work as "not always face-to-face, live sessions. It's not done in live time, the majority of it. Some of it is, but the majority is texting back and forth, [through] messaging." She explained the process of working on the platform as follows:

> What happens is there's a video that all the therapists have of ourselves, introducing ourselves. There's a matching team of people that the patient first has contact with, so that matching therapist finds out what they're looking for, what their issue is, and they provide three therapists to them to choose from. . . . they keep doing that until they find someone they like. Then I get notified via email and text that I have a new patient waiting, and I go into the [virtual] room. There are separate rooms for each patient. On my phone there's a special app that's all HIPAA compliant and encrypted. I go into the app. I find my new patient. I can leave an audio [message]. I can leave a text message in there. I give them my informed consent to sign, my emergency contact information, basically all the forms I would give my teletherapy patients. There's assessments I can give for anxiety and depression to assess on a weekly, or biweekly, basis. I introduce myself. Usually I leave audios because I think it's better. They can get my personality better, my tone. And that's how it starts. And I ask them, what brought you to treatment? I give them a little background about me

> and ask, do you have any questions about me? So, it's a little back and forth. . . . It's not about how many messages they leave. They can leave as many as they want. It's up to me to check the app once or twice a day, depending on their plan. It's whatever time I want, so I have complete flexibility. So, ten in the morning or ten o'clock at night, I can go into the room any time I want and see, okay, did anyone leave me a message? If they did, I respond. If they didn't, I don't. If they happen to respond after I check the room, they have to wait until the next day for me to check it. They can pay for live sessions. Say, for example, I'm like, listen, this is getting a little bit much. What do you think about having a live session? I'll send them a little link. They'll click on it and they'll buy a live session for thirty minutes and we will do a face-to-face, real time session in that way.

Claire described the platform itself as "amazing, innovative, [and] really reaching a lot of people." Yet this required a shift in her own thinking about what constitutes quality mental healthcare. "Look," she shared,

> I have my degree from one of the top psychoanalytic institutes in the country. Did I have some reservations about doing messaging treatment? Of course. I was like, really? This isn't treatment. You know, I was very hesitant to do it. But then working with the platform, and seeing the support that they give their therapists, and the training that they offer, and the camaraderie, and the communication between therapists, it's amazing. . . . It's actually fed me.

One of the significant differences between corporate platform-based teletherapy and independent teletherapy is that the former renders mental healthcare professionals themselves more markedly invisible than the latter. Whereas receiving screen-based treatment may result in a sense of depersonalization about healthcare providers, which Paula's earlier comments reflected, corporate platforms that offer therapy on demand and asynchronously exacerbate the dehumanization and invisibility of their workforce.

This invisibility, by extension, has serious sociocultural implications, and transforms mental healthcare providers more explicitly into gig workers.

Consider BetterHelp, a teletherapy platform that connects mental healthcare providers to persons in need, and which contains a notable clause on its informational web page for prospective employees: "Counselors are not BetterHelp employees but independent providers."[27] A similar platform, Talkspace, also considers its employees contractors and, as such, they also do not receive the protections or benefits of full-time employment. Talkspace was also the subject of investigative reporting that highlighted suspect practices related not only to patient data and privacy protections, but also its withholding of payment from therapists and policies preventing them from filing police reports. Just as Uber shifts responsibility from itself as a corporation onto its independent contractors, so too do teletherapy platforms. As journalist Cat Ferguson noted in her description of Talkspace, the company "acts like a medical provider, but its contracts and terms of use show the company acting more like a platform, passing many of the legal responsibilities of being a provider onto workers."[28]

Rationalizing Other Risks

For teletherapists who do work independently, there are a number of risks associated with practicing online that should be taken into consideration. These include unclear oversight mechanisms and regulations related to practicing in various states and countries, determining what certifications they should possess (if any) to credential themselves as teletherapists, and maintaining proficiency in ascertaining potential clients' levels of mental distress. Laura, for example, who provides teletherapy only to persons in states where she is licensed, also places great emphasis upon assessing the overall mental healthiness of prospective clients:

> So, in my office, anybody can come into my office, and as long as I can treat them, I can treat them. Whereas in e-therapy if the severity is too severe, symptoms are too severe, or they aren't old enough or can't figure things out on their own, their

> abilities aren't as strong as a teenager or somebody a little bit older, you just kind of have to be aware who it's going to work for. So if somebody's suicidal, really depressed, and they're not leaving their house, e-therapy might be a great way to start and get their foot in the door, but I would refer them to a psychiatrist or somebody in their area to get them more help and more face-to-face [therapy] because that's a little more dangerous if you don't see them face-to-face. So, I think that for some things like that you just have to be conscious of it.

Eleanor, like Laura, is licensed to practice in multiple states and provides teletherapy services to persons located in those places. She believes that multistate licensure is important for practitioners in order to ensure continuity of care, particularly when working with populations who travel often for school or for work. Although she dislikes that teletherapists are not supposed to practice over state lines, she still follows those guidelines nonetheless:

> The one gripe that I have is that we can't practice across state lines. The problem with that is that if a person goes somewhere, or lives six months out of the year somewhere, I can't counsel you where you are, [and] you need to find a new therapist for six months. . . . To find a therapist you love, and then you've got to move or whatever, it can be really limiting. So, I know a lot of therapists who will do that [for] continuity of care because, frankly, it benefits the client more than the risk that you're practicing across state lines because your client has to be somewhere else.

Yet other interviewees, including Jeremy, believe that state and national boundaries are of little importance. As noted earlier, his primary concern in determining who is a suitable international client is the degree of their mental distress. Jeremy emphasized to me that his background and skills make him adept at making determinations of who teletherapy is suited for, and responded to my questions about the ethics of practicing across borders with the following justifications:

> On a daily basis [in my other jobs] I'm screening people, evaluating people, to see if they need inpatient hospitalization. In my state I'm also a certified prescreener to screen people to see if they need to be placed under a temporary detention order. . . . I also have training to do forensic psychology evaluations, competency to stand trial evaluations. . . . Even in graduate school I was a psychology aide conducting IQ testing, different [types of] psychology testing. So that's one thing where, when I'm first going to start working with someone, I do a very thorough evaluation to see if they're going to be the right fit for it. . . . If I feel like they are, then I go ahead. If I don't, then I look for resources nearby and refer them out.

Jeremy elaborated further with more reasons he works with international clients:

> A lot of foreign countries, they don't have licensure for psychology or therapy. It's just more of a United States concept. . . . I'm not a citizen of that country and I'm not even in that country, so I'm not even sure if I have to follow their laws and regulations, and also I'm not doing any harm if I feel confident. So, when I choose the right person, I'm assessing them. I'm looking at, what are their symptoms? What are some of the safety concerns? Making a safety plan with them about whatever's going on. Looking at cultural issues as well. So, the woman I was working with [whom I mentioned earlier], she spoke English fluently. [We] didn't have a lot of cultural differences and so, you know, it worked out fine. . . . I felt like she was very low risk of, you know, harming herself or doing anything reckless. I felt like there wasn't much of a cultural barrier, so I think it worked out well.

George's reasons for practicing internationally were similar to Jeremy's:

> One reason that online therapy has been a grey area is the regulation, or lack thereof. Issues about practicing across state

> lines and things like that. I'm from the Wild West. When I was doing it [at first] there was nothing. I just learned it all, and I did it. Now I face certain risks if I get a patient who calls from Europe or something, and they want online therapy. There are some things I am doing that wouldn't be considered what you would want to be doing with online therapy, as far as things like, do you know where their local hospital is, for instance, in case they need to be hospitalized? Can I certify that they are who they say they are? Am I certified to even practice in that country? Do I have to call it something other than therapy, like coaching or something, and do another treatment? I would probably say I'm one of the few doing international [online therapy], now that I think about it. Some of these newer companies and platforms are trying it, but because of issues with the law and HIPAA and so on, they're just not taking the risk. And I'm on a couple of them that are in Europe, and the only reason I'm on them is because they know I'm experienced. Otherwise I wouldn't be on them, is what they said, because of the grey areas of international [practice]. State boundaries, same thing. I have patients in almost every state, and that means taking certain risks. I don't do it unless I know it's the right choice for the patient. They just need online [therapy], and they can't find a therapist where they live. They can't find a therapist that's as experienced as I am. [There are] many reasons that people use online therapy. So, all those things have to be evaluated.

Interviewees' feelings about the necessity of certification and training for teletherapists also varied. Jeremy sought certification as a distance credentialed counselor, noting that "it gives me confidence in what I'm doing. I don't know how many other people are getting it, but I think it's probably going to become more common." George believes that training is necessary although, as noted earlier, he is self-taught. Nonetheless he emphasized that he does not

> think anybody should be practicing online unless they have had coursework, just like any kind of license, coursework, and

> practice experience. A lot of practitioners think that because they've had phone sessions with patients, they are qualified to do online therapy, but it's totally different. Everything is different. In terms of clinically, not having them in the office. Structurally, how it's worked out. Functionally, how you work with technology. The legal and ethical issues. I believe somebody shouldn't be practicing until they have some type of that [training].

Sonja explained that even though certifications for teletherapy exist she has

> never been enamored of them. . . . I don't trust that stuff right now. I use the standards of my [state's] professional board. That I trust. . . . But there is not, that I know of, a certification that is thought well of and that is ubiquitous all over the United States. If there was something that I thought was good, or that APA thought was good, then I would [do it].

She did appreciate the training she received, however, from the internet platform that hosts her web-based sessions, although that training related only to the technical dimensions of providing screen-based therapy:

> They talked about how the shadows can block the clients from seeing your face, and how you want to be careful with glasses. . . . Where the camera is on the computer makes a big difference in what the patient perceives of the therapist. . . . If the camera is very high, like slanted, and you're looking up to the camera, that's odd and it isn't very therapeutic. But if the camera, if you set the laptop on a footstool or a side table with it low and you're in a big chair, then the camera is below you and then it's like the patient is like two feet shorter than you are. So, they really helped us. It was a one-on-one hour session with them for free.

Yet another risk that teletherapists must accept is that working in screen-based modalities might negatively affect their peers' perceptions of them as competent mental healthcare providers. Sonja shared that she has "been lectured to, certainly, that [teletherapy is] inappropriate, unethical, and so on. . . . I would say the majority of the people that I know either think it's unethical or would never do it." When I asked other interviewees whether they had received teletherapy training in school, or if it had been discussed whatsoever, affirmative answers were few and far between. Michelle told me that, during her education, all discussions of teletherapy were limited to the problems it could create:

> It was kind of like well, you know, it's harder for maintaining confidentiality to an extent, because you have to make sure that everything is done in a secured network. . . . A lot of the struggles they told us were like, you don't have that personal interaction with people, and stuff like you're not in the room with them so they may not feel as comfortable. They may not feel, you may not feel, connected to them. . . . But it wasn't covered aside from that.

Teletherapy constitutes a medical service, but that service is also understood as a social good. To reiterate Paula's assessment, those who provide teletherapy do so because they "really care at their own expense" about others, not because they anticipate that the work will be lucrative. However, even work that is motivated by altruism is, at its core, still work. Unlike other forms of care work that are necessary yet unpaid in capitalist economies, such as that which is produced within the domestic sphere,[29] teletherapists provide labor that is recognized as deserving monetary payment. To what degree and in what amount, however, are matters complicated by the indirect "compensation" that teletherapists claim their work provides: flexibility and entrepreneurialism. These are appeals that are characteristic of contemporary neoliberal economies, wherein workers come to accept economic uncertainty and precarity due to perceived immaterial benefits.

Those who professionalize themselves as teletherapists are not only gig workers, whom in exchange for flexibility accept exploitative working conditions (such as around-the-clock appointments and inadequate pay for their services), they are also rendered largely invisible workers. Again, according to Paula, patients enjoy that teletherapy lends itself to depersonalization, and they forget that they are "talking to a real person" when interacting with providers on a screen. Although the invisibility of workforces is not unique to gig economy participants, gig workers might best be understood as "more invisible" than domestic workers, for example,

> because they operate in a new fashion and through new technologies, something that is not normally associated with invisible work. Another serious risk is that the fact work is "supplied" through IT channels, being them online platforms or apps that match the demand and offer of physical chores, can "distort" the perception businesses and customers may have of these workers and significantly contribute to a perceived dehumanization of their activity.[30]

With that said, however, I believe that widespread acceptance of teletherapy transpired during the spring of 2020, a change that was borne out of necessity. The global COVID-19 pandemic legitimized screen-based medical care across a variety of domains, including those related to mental health. Nonetheless, further inquiry is needed to explore whether teletherapy's legitimation will be permanent or is only temporary, based upon exigency and emergent need.

Although I cannot speak to those questions, I can share my own experiences as a (reluctant) utilizer of teletherapy during the COVID-19 pandemic. While away from home, under a stay-at-home order, and with an appointment with my own psychologist nearing, my intent that spring had been to cancel our upcoming session. At that point this book was in its final stages of being written and, after years of thinking about teletherapy, I had concluded that it was not a therapeutic modality that I had any interest in. Even my psychologist herself was aware of my feelings. Years earlier, when we had started working together, I had been a graduate student, researching, studying, and writing the material that would one day become this book. After telling her about the fieldwork and interviews involved in my analysis of teletherapy, I remember asking if she had ever, or might ever, offer her services online. No, she had responded, she did not offer teletherapy and had no plans to.

About a week before my April 2020 appointment, therefore, I was unsure if our therapeutic relationship would be able to continue. I did not want to have a face-to-face session and did not know if my psychologist had reconsidered her own position on teletherapy. I decided to send the following email:

> Hi [name redacted],
>
> I hope that you and your family are healthy.
>
> I am emailing to actually cancel our April 6th appointment.
>
> I know you don't usually do teletherapy, but are you considering offering it due to COVID? I don't want to just like, cancel my sessions with you indefinitely, but I'm really not sure how to reschedule either.
>
> Best wishes,
> Emma

I was surprised when my psychologist quickly emailed me back to let me know that she was, in fact, now offering HIPAA-compliant teletherapy sessions. I imagined that she, like many other mental health professionals who had been critical of teletherapy in pre-COVID-19 times, had come to the conclusion that continuity of care for patients was their professional priority, regardless of their feelings about delivering care via a screen.

We rescheduled my appointment for the following week, but my trepidations about teletherapy continued to increase. I had made the deliberate choice never to seek screen-based mental healthcare for the same reasons that I never took an online class as a college student. The difference in modality, I had always believed, would significantly undermine the experience. Just as online teaching requires new pedagogical choices by instructors, and new learning habits from students, so too I imagined that teletherapy would require new cognitive strategies as a patient. Yet I already felt overwhelmed and unsure if I could muster the energy to "relearn" how to receive psychological treatment and care delivered through a screen. I had lost my job due to COVID-19-related budget cuts; I was quarantined with extended family, providing childcare and essentially homeschooling while also finishing teaching my course load for the semester. Overall, I was deeply afraid for what the future would hold for me, my family, and the world. My thoughts about teletherapy were no longer a game of hypotheticals or exercises in reflexivity and self-examination, which is what they had always been during the writing and revision processes for this book. Now teletherapy was something I was going to do in real life, not as an experiment, but because it was the only way I could actually access my mental healthcare provider.

I will readily admit that I did not enjoy teletherapy. What my psychologist and I discussed, and how we discussed it, was altogether familiar and the same as our in-person sessions. Yet doing so through a screen felt diluted, depersonalized, and even surreal when compared to my experiences sitting in her office. Yes, I had *seen* my psychologist, but it had not been face-to-face. I had watched an image of her on my screen, and that image had conversed with me, asked me questions, and responded to me. Yet the lack of spatial proximity made everything feel somehow less intimate, personal, and real. While "seeing" my psychologist offered some semblance of normalcy, it remained a poor facsimile of normalcy nonetheless.

The COVID-19 pandemic demonstrated that if we truly care about reducing health disparities, we must also accept that technological accessibility and usability need to be considered primary determinants of who has access to safe (that is, screen-based) medical care and who does not. In the context of a pandemic, for example, those without requisite technologies must choose between receiving services in-person (and risking their safety) or forgoing them entirely. In the introduction to this book I emphasized that this research, while about mental health's technologization and relationship to neoliberalism, is also about more than that. This book also presents a study of (in-)equity, (in-)justice, and the roles of various technologies in determining whose lives matter and whose do not. In the wake of COVID-19 we are no longer able to dismiss the digital divide as unimportant; technologies are literal lifelines.

This chapter began by addressing how and why teletherapy's advocates claim that telemental healthcare services increase access to quality mental healthcare. Through a combination of fieldwork and interview data, however, I have demonstrated that their claims are largely unfounded. Persons who utilize teletherapy, including me, are representative of the populations that already seek and receive the highest levels of mental healthcare services. Aside from niche populations (such as persons who travel internationally), telemental healthcare is for those whose mental distress levels are low. We are not representative of persons or populations whose need for mental healthcare services have been underserved, historically or today.

Teletherapy might facilitate the elimination of some barriers to accessing mental healthcare services, such as an inability to schedule sessions during work hours or ongoing childcare responsibilities. Alternatively it may be a preferable therapeutic modality, as Michelle stated is the case for persons unable to leave their homes but who also do not want visitors inside them. Nonetheless, teletherapy's promise to increase access to mental healthcare remains largely unsubstantiated. While teletherapy increases the quality of care patients receive, those who are already motivated enough to seek out mental healthcare services will likely do so regardless of whether it is via a screen or face-to-face. Screen-based therapy, for most of those who choose to utilize those services, are not the only way that mental healthcare can be accessed; it is simply the most convenient. Convenience, however, is a matter separate and distinct from accessibility. Accessibility must account as well for justice and equity.[31]

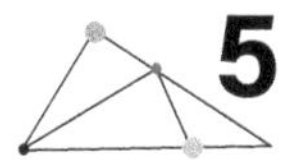

5

The Future of Mental Health Technologies

Polly[1] is the director of a midsized residential facility for adults with severe, persistent mental illnesses, personality disorders, and brain injuries. All of her residents require high levels of care, and all are on Social Security. "They don't work, and they don't have a lot of money. They have $97 a month," she explained to me. I had recruited Polly for an interview to discuss her perceptions of mental health technologies, particularly whether they might be beneficial to high-needs individuals like her residents. While on a few occasions, she shared, virtual visits with doctors had been useful for a handful of residents, she doubted that any technology could ever satisfy their healthcare needs: "A lot of [the residents] have a cellphone, but it's kind of a basic cellphone. Some have smartphones, but they're not the most advanced phones. Our residents don't really have a strong grasp of technology, beyond the basic. They can go on Facebook, they might have an email address, but for the most part they communicate face-to-face in the wider world." As to who would find smartphone applications, teletherapy, or therapeutic chatbots useful, Polly predicted it would have to be "somebody who has more advanced social skills. . . . They don't need the twenty-four-hour support that our clients need. They can manage their day-to-day lives. They just need a little extra support."

I share this information about Polly and her residents to highlight the incongruity between how proponents of mental health technologies imagine their utility and what their practical limits truly are. Throughout this book I have demonstrated that advocates of smartphone applications, algorithms, AI chatbots, and teletherapy believe that technologies make mental healthcare more accessible. In actuality, however, they do not. "Access" is not just a matter of tools or technologies existing; to truly increase access, technologies must also be obtainable and usable by persons who want or need them, lead to positive health outcomes, and reduce existing healthcare disparities. Simply creating a technology and claiming that, by the very nature of its being, it increases the accessibility of healthcare services does not make that claim true. Yet operating under such a premise allows technologists, healthcare professionals, and other invested parties to justify directing immense resources toward the development of new technologies when, in fact, those resources could be put to much better use elsewhere.

In the conference fieldwork and interviews presented throughout this book, I witnessed and heard the ways in which those justifications transpire. Many of those whom I interacted with, or whose presentations and speeches I saw, seemed to genuinely believe that their work has positive social, cultural, and medical effects. They are not entirely wrong. Smartphone applications, therapeutic chatbots, teletherapy, and even psychosurveillance have the ability to improve continuums of existing care, and may also be beneficial to subclinical populations. Yet Polly's suggestion that mental health technologies are most useful for persons who "just need a little extra support" was incredibly apt, as these technologies are not making mental healthcare accessible to already underserved populations whose needs continue to go unmet. Those who advocate for mental health's technologization, whether intentionally or not, are disregarding those populations' needs in pursuit of an easier task: improving the quality of care for persons already possessing the requisite tools and resources to obtain mental healthcare services in the first place.

Technology cannot solve the ongoing mental healthcare crisis, nor can it solve any other problem or crisis. Technology is not a panacea. The desire to implement technologies in new and exciting ways, even to improve social, cultural, or medical problems, more so reflects our dreams and aspirations about technologies' capabilities than it does their actual usefulness. Technologies may mask inequity and disparity, at least temporarily, but will ultimately only perpetuate the systemic problems that pre-dated them. A more productive approach would be to address the social, cultural, and historical problems and contexts that lead us to dream of technological solutions to crises, including the mental healthcare crisis, in the first place. This would involve commitment to interrogating and eradicating discriminatory and prejudiced beliefs and practices, including racism, classism, and sexism, which are intrinsically interwoven into the domains of both medicine and technology. We must also dispel the belief that medicine and technology are apolitical, value-neutral, and objective in their own conceptualizations and treatments of bodies. There is no possibility of creating "neutral" health technologies, as neither medicine nor technology are "neutral" unto themselves.

In chapter 1 of this book I argued that smartphone applications, created for the purposes of improving user mental health, are emblematic of the neoliberal ethos of responsibilization. Yet by exploring whose responsibilization they are intended to enhance, it became clear that they not only perpetuate white prototypicality,[2] but also that they are meant for a demographic that is predominantly young and female. Their design may feel "neutral" to the creators of these technologies, yet they are fundamentally political, reflecting beliefs about who should be provided the opportunity to engage in technologically facilitated regimes of health practices and whose exclusion from participation is justified.

Chapter 2 explored the emergence of psychosurveillance and its deployment as a form of communitarian labor on platforms such as Facebook, 7 Cups of Tea, and Crisis Text Line. While technologies may promise to empower their users, even in domains related to mental health, they ultimately enhance our responsibilization capacities and, in turn, demand new modes of labor. Rather than strive for structural solutions to the mental healthcare crisis, each of us is held accountable for the monitoring and management of others' mental and emotional states in online contexts. This results in a spectrum of exploitative labor practices for those who volunteer as psychosurveillance providers, either informally on social media or explicitly on platforms like 7 Cups of Tea and Crisis Text Line.

This book's third chapter examined a number of therapeutic

chatbots made possible by artificial intelligence. Yet they, perhaps even more so than smartphone applications, reify a technological imaginary that systematically excludes persons who are in the highest need of mental healthcare resources, particularly people of color.[3] Rather than expand the accessibility of those services, these tools articulate the bodies of persons in need as, again, young and white.

Finally, chapter 4 examined how a technologized modality of care (that being screen-based mental healthcare services) has transformed practices and beliefs about the economic and social value of mental healthcare itself. By analyzing my conversations with teletherapists, I demonstrated how they—as workers—are encouraged to appropriate professional and financial risks associated with neoliberal entrepreneurialism. They, like app developers, often believe that teletherapy increases the accessibility of mental healthcare resources, although my analysis demonstrates that their work improves continuums of care without increasing access to care.

If we are truly and genuinely invested in increasing access to mental healthcare services, then it is clear from the findings presented in this book that technologies are in no way capable of facilitating necessary changes. I am therefore calling for a turn away from technological solutionism in the domain of mental health, and instead urging that we redirect resources toward recruiting and training culturally competent mental health professionals to provide the healthcare services that are so sorely needed in the United States and across the globe. Through a combination of legislative initiatives and demands for change and justice, I believe that such a future might come to fruition.

Yet while those are my hopes, I worry that perhaps my fears are more realistic: a future wherein we are no longer merely encouraged to turn toward mental health technologies in the name of responsibilization but are instead explicitly forced to do so, not only due to an inability to repair a broken healthcare system, but also in the name of public health and safety. Consider a series of remarks given in August 2019 by President Donald Trump, as he offered condolences to the victims of mass shootings in El Paso, Texas, and Dayton, Ohio. Although his speech began with the usual offerings of thoughts and prayers, those remarks soon took a turn:

> We must shine light on the dark recesses of the Internet, and stop mass murders before they start. The Internet, likewise, is used for human trafficking, illegal drug distribution, and so many other heinous crimes. The perils of the Internet and social media cannot be ignored, and they will not be ignored. . . . First, we must do a better job of identifying and acting on early warning signs. I am directing the Department of Justice to work in partisan—partnership with local, state, and federal agencies, as well as social media companies, to develop tools that can detect mass shooters before they strike. As an example, the monster in the Parkland high school in Florida had many red flags against him, and yet nobody took decisive action. Nobody did anything. Why not?[4]

While blaming "the internet" or other technologies is not unusual in the midst of a moral panic,[5] Trump's suggestion contained a notable clause: that we should be using technology (he referred repeatedly to the internet) to prevent crime and "stop mass murders before they start." *Was such a world possible?*, many of us began to ask ourselves. *A world where the internet and social media could be harnessed to prevent crime?* In turn Marisa Randazzo, the U.S. Secret Service's former chief research psychologist, told the *Washington Post* that "there's so many things about this idea of predicting violence that doesn't make sense": "Even if the technology could be developed, such a program would probably flag tens, or hundreds of thousands, more possible suspects than actual shooters. How, she asked, would you sort through them? And how would you know you were right, given the difficulty of proving something that hasn't happened?"[6]

On the one hand, perhaps omnipresent mental health monitoring and surveillance, facilitated by an array of technologies including social media algorithms and wearable devices capable of digital phenotyping, might normalize and destigmatize mental distress and illness. My concern, however, is that whatever data is produced will be used to deny us our civil liberties, laying the groundwork for discrimination based upon presumptions about our mental health and aptitudes or predispositions for violence based on the medicalization of collected information. I do not want to live in such a world, wherein mental health data is not only manufactured by technologies but also utilized for explicitly political purposes. Yet technologies cannot be divested from the contexts in which they emerge, as cultural forces and imperatives play pivotal roles in their development and deployment. If they are created in the context of fear and motivated by an ethos of prevention, as Trump himself suggested, then their implementation will likely exacerbate inequalities. I fear that despite this knowledge, many of us will still come to believe that accepting further social, cultural, and medical stratification is a necessary part of keeping us safe.

Returning to the present moment, we do not yet live in such a world. The world that we do inhabit, however, is one thoroughly enmeshed with neoliberal values, and the technologies I have analyzed and discussed throughout this book reflect some of governmentality's multiform tactics as well as our internalization of the individuation of responsibility. As responsible citizenship practices are made possible through the use of technologies that act as mechanisms of control and oversight, their utilization also signals the death of health, even mental health, as a private and individual matter, and instead positions an individual's willingness to share that information as emblematic of communitarianism. Randazzo was clear that there is no predictive technology capable of providing what Trump seemingly called for: a way to determine which persons with mental illnesses will carry out acts of violence. Even so, the argument that we must forfeit privacy and accept mental health technologies as part of our normative regimes of self-care, I predict, will manifest soon, as psychosurveillance becomes increasingly framed as the only way to inoculate ourselves from the "threat" of mentally ill persons, a belief perpetuated by many discourses circulating in response to an epidemic of mass shootings and violence.[7]

Already mental health technologies function as apparatuses of social control, despite not (yet) being explicitly weaponized in violence prevention. They promote and reflect a particular vision of social order, one that in its ideal form would be devoid of mental illness and disorder. While on its face striving to eliminate mental illness might seem uncontroversial, there is a fine line between health promotion and the pursuit of a eugenicist agenda, a possibility that speaks to the concerns and predictions of neurodiversity activists and scholars alike.[8]

I would have liked to conclude this book on a more positive note, not to have felt compelled to offer so bleak a prediction of how mental health technologies might intersect with social and political imperatives and practices in the future. Yet I choose to share that imagined future with you because our goal should be to prevent such a world from being realized. With that in mind, the information presented in this book has sought to speak to multiple audiences: those who are curious about the role of technology in the delivery of healthcare, those with interest in the ethical dimensions of digital health and healthcare disparities, healthcare policy makers, healthcare workers, technologists and software designers, data scientists and other researchers, and members of the general public who have ever used mental health technologies or are considering them. All of us can work together in pursuit of a more just future.

Of course, the challenge in studying a technology, or technologies, is that by the time the research goes to print, the topics discussed or tool sets analyzed may be obsolete. Although the particularized objects of my analysis will (inevitably) someday be outdated, the claims and arguments that I have made about the relationships between mental health technologies, social control, and their relationships to and with medicine will remain the same.

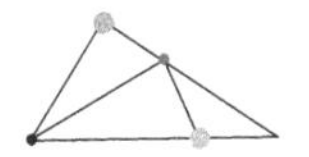

COVID Coda

Widespread technological dependency increased exponentially during the spring of 2020 as COVID-19 spread across the globe. For many, computers, smart devices, and internet connectivity became necessary for physical safety, as they facilitated the ability to work from home, attend school remotely, and seek and receive medical care. In fact, roughly 53 percent of U.S. adults came to describe the internet as "essential" in the midst of the pandemic.[1]

Yet prior to the pandemic, research had already established persistent and ongoing disparities related not only to technological access but also to health. Persons who were nonwhite, geographically remote, less educated, and with lower incomes were already less likely to have computers, smart technologies, and internet at home.[2] We also knew that those who identify as Black, African American, Hispanic, and Latino were far more likely than white and Asian Americans to be employed in service jobs, work that could not be performed remotely and that, by extension, would increase their likelihood of exposure to coronavirus.[3]

With the health of the U.S. population in mind, in March 2020 the Department of Health and Human Services decided to relax its guidelines, releasing a statement that it would no longer penalize healthcare providers unable to be HIPAA compliant while providing medical services. Now healthcare professionals could "see" their patients via the previously forbidden platforms of Skype, FaceTime, and Google Hangouts.[4] Also in the name of increasing access to safe medical services, more and more medical offices and hospitals turned to telemedicine to prevent the spread of the virus.[5]

Despite those changes, there was no systematic attempt to address the needs of persons without insurance, in high-risk occupations, and without internet and technological access at home. Although we already knew that persons without medical insurance were more likely to come from low-income families and to be nonwhite,[6] and that Black Americans in particular had disproportionately low insurance coverage,[7] no concrete steps were taken to reduce those disparities. Instead, during the summer of 2020, the Centers for Disease Control only offered the following statement:

> Long-standing systemic health and social inequities have put many people from racial and ethnic minority groups at increased risk of getting sick and dying from COVID-19. . . . Social determinants of health have historically prevented them from having fair opportunities for economic, physical, and emotional health.
>
> There is increasing evidence that some racial and ethnic minority groups are being disproportionately affected by COVID-19. Inequities in the social determinants of health, such as poverty and healthcare access, affecting these groups are interrelated and influence a wide range of health and quality-of-life outcomes and risks. To achieve health equity, barriers must be removed so that everyone has a fair opportunity to be as healthy as possible.[8]

While there was now agreement that COVID-19's effects were amplified among already-marginalized populations, there was significantly less discourse about the relationships between technological access, socioeconomic status, and mental health during the pandemic.

Generally speaking, COVID-19 had caused the landscape of mental healthcare services and systems to change. Prior to the pandemic, thirty-one million Americans (roughly one in eleven people) relied upon community health clinics for medical care, including mental healthcare. Those resources dissipated, however, as the virus caused many such clinics to shutter.[9] Some, who under normal circumstances would be hospitalized due to suicidal intent and ideation, were discharged from hospitals that had to make space for quarantined COVID-19 patients.[10] Nearly half of all adults in the United States polled in March 2020 believed that COVID-19 was negatively impacting their mental health,[11] and, as the pandemic surged, so too did calls to the National Alliance on Mental Illness's HelpLine and similar hotlines.[12] Mental healthcare professionals noted the increase in demand for their services,[13] and many internet-based mental health platforms and applications experienced rapid growth.[14]

In addition to changes in the here-and-now, dire predictions began to emerge about the likely long-term, negative mental health effects of the pandemic. We were told that essential and front-line workers would one day experience unprecedentedly high rates of anxiety, depression, stress, and post-traumatic stress disorders as a result of the pandemic.[15] There was even clinical research to suggest that COVID-19 itself causes changes to brain function and structure.[16] In May 2020 the United Nations issued a policy brief titled "COVID-19 and the Need for Action on Mental Health," not only detailing what was known about the virus's effects upon mental health and cognitive functioning but also advocating for robust mental health reform to prevent further suffering.

In August 2020, the Centers for Disease Control published the results of a study titled "Mental Health, Substance Use, and Suicidal Ideation During the COVID-19 Pandemic," which included a particularly notable sentence: "Mental health conditions are disproportionately affecting specific populations, especially young adults, Hispanic persons, black persons, essential workers, unpaid caregivers for adults, and those receiving treatment for preexisting psychiatric conditions."[17] Yet even in its own affirmation of the results of the study, the Substance Abuse and Mental Health Services Administration spoke in generalities, noting that the findings were

> troubling but unfortunately not surprising. The Assistant Secretary for Mental Health and Substance Use, Dr. Elinore McCance-Katz, has warned of the emergence of increased mental health and substance use issues since the start of the pandemic. . . . The Assistant Secretary again urges local and state officials to consider all aspects of health and not solely

> virus containment as we move forward. Research is clear on the effect of shutdown and social isolation on an individual's mental health. The negative health effects are potentially long-lasting and very consequential for individuals and their families. . . . We cannot continue to ignore the health consequences for all other conditions in favor of singularly focusing on virus containment.[18]

There was no indication that the pressing needs of people of color, whose risk of mental distress was compounded by socioeconomic status, type of employment, and technological inequity, were of particular concern to any government entity whatsoever.

Instead, neoliberalism's emphasis upon the individuation of responsibility in lieu of implementing systemic support mechanisms led us to believe that if changes would come, they would result from private initiatives. Enter the Boris Lawrence Henson Foundation, a nonprofit organization spearheaded by Taraji P. Henson. While the foundation's initial aim was to destigmatize mental healthcare services in the African American population, its focus shifted during the pandemic:

> Given the life-changing events related to or triggered by the COVID-19 pandemic, many are suffering in silence and isolation. The Boris L. Henson Foundation (BLHF) recognizes that during this difficult time, affording the cost of mental health services can be a barrier in the African-American community. Having to choose between a meal and mental health is not something that one should ever have to ponder. . . . Individuals with life-changing stressors and anxiety related to the coronavirus will have the cost for up to five (5) individual sessions defrayed on a first come, first serve basis until all funds are committed or exhausted.[19]

Henson's efforts were praised by publications and news outlets including the *Washington Post*,[20] *NBC News*,[21] *Essence*,[22] and more. Certainly, those accolades were much deserved.

Yet in our acknowledgment and appreciation of what Henson and the Boris Lawrence Henson Foundation provided and accomplished, we run the risk of forgetting that another world and future is possible. In that future we would not have to rely upon the generosity of private actors to address the health and technological disparities that are now more pronounced than ever. Instead, just and equitable access to healthcare services would involve consideration of the role of technology in making health practices possible. If, in the midst of the COVID-19 pandemic, the safest option for mental healthcare is for it to be delivered via a screen, so be it, despite the critiques and criticisms I have previously offered in my analysis of teletherapy.[23] Mental healthcare must be made accessible, and if a global pandemic precludes that care from being provided face-to-face, screen-based services will have to do—for now. As the pandemic has shown us, technologies are lifelines that make it possible to safely access medical care without risking illness. If we accept teletherapy, we must accept responsibility for eliminating digital divides. To do one without the other will only further exacerbate inequalities.

When technologies are neither accessible nor usable by all of us, equally, they have no place as determinants of who can and cannot access healthcare services.

Another world is possible.

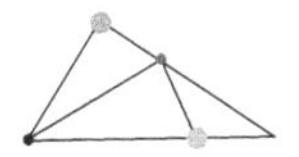

Acknowledgments

I am not sure this book would have been completed without the love, support, and patience of two people in particular: my husband, Alexander, and my mother, Roberta. Other members of my family, including my sister, Gabrielle, and nephews Mason and Maxwell, have also been my champions throughout the writing (and rewriting, and rewriting . . .) process. Copper, you are also an endless source of cuddles and kisses.

Throughout my life I have been fortunate to meet and learn from many scholars and teachers who played formative roles in my own development as a thinker, writer, and educator. These include (in the order in which we met) Atsushi Tajima, Laurie Ouellette, and Carl Elliott. Thank you as well to Ron Greene and Catherine Squires, both of whom served on my dissertation committee, and to Tony Lin.

The University of Minnesota provided me with immense support as a graduate student, not only in my home department of communication studies, but also in the forms of an Interdisciplinary Doctoral Fellowship through the Center for Bioethics and a Critical Data Studies Fellowship through the Informatics Institute. With their funding I was able to conduct many of the interviews and much of the fieldwork involved in this research.

Finally, I must extend my sincerest thanks to the University of Minnesota Press and my editor, Leah Pennywark. She believed in this work at a time when I was losing hope that anyone might ever think it had value. Due to her insight and guidance, *Therapy*

Tech has become a book that I am proud to have written. Thank you as well to all others who had a hand in the writing, editing, and production of this book: Anne Carter, Wendy Holdman, Ana Bichanich, Martyn Schmoll, Kristine Hunt, and the reviewers who provided me with invaluable feedback on earlier versions of this manuscript.

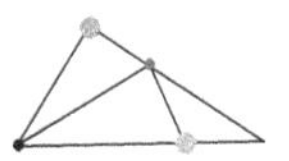

Notes

Introduction

1. John M. Kane, "Comments on Abilify MyCite," *Clinical Schizophrenia & Related Psychoses* 11, no. 4 (2018): 205–6; Lisa Rosenbaum, "Swallowing a Spy—The Potential Uses of Digital Adherence Monitoring," *New England Journal of Medicine* 378, no. 2 (2018): 101–3.
2. "FDA Approves Pill with Sensor that Digitally Tracks If Patients Have Ingested Their Medication," Food and Drug Administration, November 13, 2017, https://www.fda.gov.
3. Pam Belluck, "First Digital Pill Approved to Worries about 'Biomedical 'Big Brother,'" *New York Times,* November 13, 2017, https://www.nytimes.com.
4. Belluck, "First Digital Pill."
5. "Mental Illness," National Institute of Mental Health, 2019, https://www.nimh.nih.gov.
6. "Learn About Mental Health," Centers for Disease Control, January 26, 2018, https://www.cdc.gov.
7. Linda Girgis, "Is There a Mental Healthcare Crisis in the US?," *Physician's Weekly,* July 29, 2014, http://www.physiciansweekly.com; David Levine, "What's the Answer to the Shortage of Mental Health Care Providers?," *U.S. News & World Report,* May 25, 2018, https://health.usnews.com.
8. Bartley Christopher Frueh, "Solving Mental Healthcare Access Problems in the Twenty-First Century," *Australian Psychologist* 50, no. 4 (2015): 304–6.
9. Kathleen Rowan, Donna D. McAlpine, and Lynn A. Blewett, "Access and Cost Barriers to Mental Health Care, by Insurance Status, 1999–2010," *Health Affairs* 32, no. 10 (2013): 1723–30.
10. Frueh, "Solving Mental Healthcare Access Problems," 304.
11. Michel Foucault, *The Birth of Biopolitics: Lectures at the Collège de France, 1978–1979,* trans. Graham Burchell, ed. Michel Senellart, Francois Ewald, Alessandro Fontana, and Arnold I. Davidson (New York: Palgrave Macmillan, 2008).

12. Kathleen LeBesco, "Neoliberalism, Public Health, and the Moral Perils of Fatness," *Critical Public Health* 21, no. 2 (2011): 153–64.
13. For examples of this scholarship see Emma Bedor, "It's Not You, It's Your (Old) Vagina: Osphena's Articulation of Sexual Dysfunction," *Sexuality & Culture* 20, no. 1 (2015): 38–55; Michelle Hannah Smirnova, "A Will to Youth: The Woman's Anti-Aging Elixir," *Social Science & Medicine* 75, no. 7 (2012): 1236–43; Kristin Swenson, *Lifestyle Drugs and the Neoliberal Family* (New York: Peter Lang, 2013).
14. Joy Fuqua, *Prescription TV: Therapeutic Discourse in the Hospital and at Home* (Durham, N.C.: Duke University Press, 2012).
15. Paul Crawshaw, "Governing the Healthy Male Citizen: Men, Masculinity and Popular Health in *Men's Health* Magazine," *Social Science & Medicine* 65 (2007): 1606–18.
16. Michel Foucault, *The Foucault Effect: Studies in Governmentality*, ed. Graham Burchell, Colin Gordon, and Peter Miller (London: Harvester Wheatsheaf, 1991).
17. Foucault, *The Foucault Effect*, 95.
18. "A Health Care App You'll Actually Use," Oscar, 2020, https://www.hioscar.com.
19. "UnitedHealthcare Motion," UnitedHealthcare, 2020, https://www.uhc.com.
20. "Vitality Program," John Hancock, 2020, https://www.johnhancock.com.
21. Bill Sherman, "Fitbit Fitness Monitoring Program a Hit at ORU," *Tulsa World*, March 20, 2017, https://www.tulsaworld.com/.
22. Edgar Alvarez, "Adidas Designed a Wearable for PE Class," *Engadget*, April 5, 2016, https://www.engadget.com.
23. For one example of this scholarship—though there are many—see Harold W. Kohl, Cora Lynn Craig, Estelle Victoria Lambert, Shigeru Inoue, Jasem Ramadan Alkandari, Grit Leetongin, and Sonja Kahlmeier, "The Pandemic of Physical Inactivity: Global Action for Public Health," *The Lancet* 380, no. 9838 (2012): 294–305.
24. Andrea H. Weinberger, Misato Gbedemah, A. M. Martinez, Denis Nash, Sandro Galea, and Renee D. Goodwin, "Trends in Depression Prevalence in the USA from 2005 to 2015: Widening Disparities in Vulnerable Groups," *Psychological Medicine* 48, no. 8 (2018): 1308–15.
25. Jean M. Twenge, A. Bell Cooper, Thomas E. Joiner, Mary E. Duffy, and Sarah G. Binau, "Age, Period, and Cohort Trends in Mood Disorder Indicators and Suicide-Related Outcomes in a Nationally Representative Dataset, 2005–2017," *Journal of Abnormal Psychology* 128, no. 3 (2019): 185–99.
26. Paul E. Greenberg, Andree-Anne Fournier, Tammy Sisitsky, Crystal T. Pike, and Ronald C. Kessler, "The Economic Burden of Adults with Major Depressive Disorder in the United States (2005 and 2010)," *Journal of Clinical Psychiatry* 76, no. 2 (2015): 155–62.

27. Kate Kelland, "Mental Health Crisis Could Cost the World $16 Trillion by 2030," *Reuters,* October 9, 2018, https://www.reuters.com.
28. Nikolas Rose, "Disorders Without Borders? The Expanding Scope of Psychiatric Practice," *BioSocieties* 1, no. 4 (2006): 474.
29. Peter Conrad, *The Medicalization of Society: On the Transformation of Human Conditions into Treatable Disorders* (Baltimore, Md.: Johns Hopkins University Press, 2007).
30. Erik Parens, "On Good and Bad Forms of Medicalization," *Bioethics* 27, no. 1 (2013): 29.
31. Allen Frances, "The Past, Present and Future of Psychiatric Diagnosis," *World Psychiatry* 12, no. 2 (2013): 111.
32. Marina Levina and Roswell Quinn, "From Symptomatic to Pre-Symptomatic Patient: The Tide of Personal Genomics," *Journal of Science Communication* 10, no. 3 (2011): C03.
33. For an early example of this claim see Kenneth Irving Zola, "Toward the Necessary Universalizing of a Disability Policy," *Milbank Quarterly* 83, no. 4 (1989): 401–28.
34. Nikolas Rose and Joelle M. Abi-Rached, *Neuro: The New Brain Sciences and the Management of the Mind* (Princeton, N.J.: Princeton University Press, 2013), 48. Italics in original.
35. Rose and Abi-Rached, *Neuro,* 52. Italics added for emphasis.
36. Dan Hurley, "Can You Make Yourself Smarter?," *New York Times,* April 18, 2012, https://www.nytimes.com/.
37. Brain training has a fascinating history. Some examples of works where it is discussed include Simon Makin, "Brain Training: Memory Games," *Nature* 531 (2016): S10–S11; Benjamin Katz, "Brain-Training Isn't Just a Modern Phenomenon, the Edwardians Were Also Fans," *The Conversation,* September 1, 2014 https://theconversation.com.
38. John Torous, Joseph Firth, Kit Huckvale, Mark E. Larsen, Theodore D. Cosco, Rebekah Carney, Steven Chan, et al., "The Emerging Imperative for a Consensus Approach toward the Rating and Clinical Recommendation of Mental Health Apps," *Journal of Nervous and Mental Disease* 206, no. 8 (2018): 662–66.
39. See examples of this work from Berna A. Sari, Ernst H. W. Koster, Gilles Pourtois, and Nazanin Derakshan, "Training Working Memory to Improve Attentional Control in Anxiety: A Proof-of-Principle Study Using Behavioral and Electrophysiological Measures," *Biological Psychology* 121 (2016): 203–12; Sabine Wanmaker, Elke Geraerts, and Ingmar H. A. Franken, "A Working Memory Training to Decrease Rumination in Depressed and Anxious Individuals: A Double-Blind Randomized Controlled Trial," *Journal of Affective Disorders* 175 (2015): 310–19.
40. In media and cultural studies this framing is often attributed to the work of Laurie Ouellette and James Hay, particularly in relation to the cultural function of reality television. See Laurie Ouellette and

James Hay, "Makeover Television, Governmentality and the Good Citizen," *Continuum* 22, no. 4 (2008): 471–84.

41. Deborah Lupton, "Critical Perspectives on Digital Health Technologies," *Sociology Compass* 8, no. 12 (2014): 1344–45.
42. There is often confusion regarding the different types of mental health professions and what the qualifications, trainings, and certifications are for each. To better understand those differences, I suggest this resource from the American Psychological Association: "What Is the Difference Between Psychologists, Psychiatrists and Social Workers?," American Psychological Association, 2017, https://www.apa.org.
43. Warren Kinghorn, "The Biopolitics of Defining 'Mental Disorder,'" in *Making the DSM-5: Concepts and Controversies*, ed. Joel Paris and James Phillips (New York: Springer, 2013), 47.
44. Brett J. Deacon, "The Biomedical Model of Mental Disorder: A Critical Analysis of its Validity, Utility, and Effects on Psychotherapy Research," *Clinical Psychology Review* 33, no. 7 (2013): 846–61.
45. For some discussion of the relationship between mental healthcare and culture see Glorisa Canino and Margarita Alegría, "Psychiatric Diagnosis—Is It Universal or Relative to Culture?," *Journal of Child Psychology and Psychiatry* 49, no. 3 (2008): 237–50; Renato D. Alarcón, "Culture, Cultural Factors and Psychiatric Diagnosis: Review and Projections," *World Psychiatry* 8, no. 3 (2009): 131; John Widdup Berry, Ype H. Poortinga, Marshall H. Segall, and Pierre R. Dasen, *Cross-Cultural Psychology: Research and Applications* (New York: Cambridge University Press, 2002).
46. Pamela A. Hays, "Multicultural Applications of Cognitive-Behavior Therapy," *Professional Psychology: Research and Practice* 26, no. 3 (1995): 309.
47. Hays, "Multicultural Applications of Cognitive-Behavior Therapy," 309.
48. Tanya M. Luhrmann, Ramachandran Padmavati, Hema Tharoor, and Akwasi Osei, "Differences in Voice-Hearing Experiences of People with Psychosis in the USA, India and Ghana: Interview-Based Study," *British Journal of Psychiatry* 206, no. 1 (2015): 42.
49. For some examples see Jack Drescher, "Queer Diagnoses: Parallels and Contrasts in the History of Homosexuality, Gender Variance, and the Diagnostic and Statistical Manual," *Archives of Sexual Behavior* 39, no. 2 (2010): 427–60; Sonia Schwartz, "The Role of Values in the Nature/Nurture Debate about Psychiatric Disorders," *Social Psychiatry and Psychiatric Epidemiology* 33, no. 8 (1998): 356–62.
50. Some scholarship in this vein includes Charlotte Brownlow, "Re-Presenting Autism: The Construction of 'NT Syndrome,'" *Journal of Medical Humanities* 31, no. 3 (2010): 243–55; Katherine Runswick-Cole, "'Us' and 'Them': The Limits and Possibilities of a 'Politics of

Neurodiversity' in Neoliberal Times," *Disability & Society* 29, no. 7 (2014): 1117–29; Brigit McWade, Damian Milton, and Peter Beresford, "Mad Studies and Neurodiversity: A Dialogue," *Disability & Society* 30, no. 2 (2015): 305–9.

51. Runswick-Cole, "'Us' and 'Them.'"
52. McWade, Milton, and Beresford, "Mad Studies and Neurodiversity," 306.
53. Schwartz, "The Role of Values in the Nature/Nurture Debate," 357.
54. Ilza Veith, *Hysteria: The History of a Disease* (Lanham, Md.: Jason Aronson, 1993); Jane M. Ussher, "A Critical Feminist Analysis of Madness: Pathologising Femininity through Psychiatric Discourse," in *Routledge International Handbook of Critical Mental Health,* ed. Bruce M. Z. Cohen (New York: Routledge, 2018), 96–102.
55. Parens, "On Good and Bad Forms of Medicalization."
56. Gary Greenberg, *The Book of Woe: The DSM and the Unmaking of Psychiatry* (New York: Blue Rider, 2013), 2.
57. Some examples of this scholarship include Rena Bivens, "The Gender Binary Will Not Be Deprogrammed: Ten Years of Coding Gender on Facebook," *New Media & Society* 19, no. 6 (2017): 880–98; Lars Z. Mackenzie, "The Afterlife of Data: Identity, Surveillance, and Capitalism in Trans Credit Reporting," *Transgender Studies Quarterly* 4, no. 1 (2017): 45–60; Anja Lambrecht and Catherine Tucker, "Algorithmic Bias? An Empirical Study of Apparent Gender-Based Discrimination in the Display of STEM Career Ads," *Management Science* 65, no. 7 (2019): 2966–81; Caroline Criado Perez, *Invisible Women: Data Bias in a World Designed for Men* (New York: Abrams, 2019).
58. See Safiya Umoja Noble, *Algorithms of Oppression: How Search Engines Reinforce Racism* (New York: New York University Press, 2018); Frank Pasquale, *The Black Box Society* (Cambridge. Mass.: Harvard University Press, 2015).
59. José van Dijck, "Datafication, Dataism and Dataveillance: Big Data between Scientific Paradigm and Ideology," *Surveillance & Society* 12, no. 2 (2014): 197–208; Mark Andrejevic and Kelly Gates, "Big Data Surveillance: Introduction," *Surveillance & Society* 12, no. 2 (2014): 185–96.
60. Olivia Banner, *Communicative Biocapitalism: The Voice of the Patient in Digital Health and the Health Humanities* (Ann Arbor: University of Michigan Press, 2017).
61. Meredith Broussard, *Artificial Unintelligence: How Computers Misunderstand the World* (Cambridge, Mass.: MIT Press, 2018); Mark Marino, "The Racial Formation of Chatbots," *CLCWeb: Comparative Literature and Culture* 16, no. 5 (2014): 13.
62. Sarah T. Roberts, *Behind the Screen: Content Moderation in the Shadows of Social Media* (New Haven, Conn.: Yale University Press,

2019); Tarleton Gillespie, *Custodians of the Internet: Platforms, Content Moderation, and the Hidden Decisions That Shape Social Media* (New Haven, Conn.: Yale University Press, 2018).

63. Ruha Benjamin, *Race After Technology: Abolitionist Tools for the New Jim Code* (New York: Polity, 2019). Discriminatory design is a long-standing interest of Dr. Benjamin's, and I am very much inspired by her work. I was fortunate to meet and learn from her when she provided a keynote at the University of Minnesota's Critical Data Studies symposium in 2016.
64. Noble, *Algorithms of Oppression.*
65. Simone Browne, "Digital Epidermalization: Race, Identity and Biometrics," *Critical Sociology* 36, no. 1 (2010): 131–50.
66. Lisa Nakamura, *Cybertypes: Race, Ethnicity, and Identity on the Internet* (New York: Routledge, 2013).
67. Judith A. Cook and Mary Margaret Fonow, "Knowledge and Women's Interests: Issues of Epistemology and Methodology in Feminist Sociological Research," *Sociological Inquiry* 56, no. 1 (1986): 2–29.
68. For discussions on this topic see Ruth Behar and Deborah A. Gordon, eds., *Women Writing Culture* (Berkeley: University of California Press, 1995); Kum-Kum Bhavnani, "Empowerment and Social Research: Some Comments," *Text—Interdisciplinary Journal for the Study of Discourse* 8, no. 1–2 (1988): 41–50; Lilliana Del Busso, "III. Embodying Feminist Politics in the Research Interview: Material Bodies and Reflexivity," *Feminism & Psychology* 17, no. 3 (2007): 309–15.
69. I received IRB approval for the interviews included in chapters 1, 4, and 5 of this book. Participation was anonymous, and any potentially identifying information was omitted or altered in final versions of transcripts. My discussions with therapeutic chatbot creators, included in chapter 3, were not anonymized. Both Alison Darcy and Danny Freed were aware that I would name them in my writings about our conversations.
70. Sara L. Crawley, "Autoethnography as Feminist Self-Interview," in *The SAGE Handbook of Interview Research: The Complexity of the Craft,* ed. Jaber F. Gubrium, James A. Holstein, Amir B. Marvasti, and Karyn D. McKinney (Thousand Oaks, Calif.: Sage, 2012): 143–61.
71. Kamala Visweswaran, *Fictions of Feminist Ethnography* (Minneapolis: University of Minnesota Press, 1994).
72. There is limited work on this area, but some examples include Christine Hine, *Virtual Ethnography* (Thousand Oaks, Calif.: Sage, 2000); Nicole Marie Brown, "Methodological Cyborg as Black Feminist Technology: Constructing the Social Self Using Computational Digital Autoethnography and Social Media," *Cultural Studies↔Critical Methodologies* 19, no. 1 (2019): 55–67; Tasha R.

Dunn and W. Benjamin Myers, "Contemporary Autoethnography Is Digital Autoethnography: A Proposal for Maintaining Methodological Relevance in Changing Times," *Journal of Autoethnography* 1, no. 1 (2020): 43–59.

73. This point is emphasized in Brown, "Methodological Cyborg," and Dunn and Myers, "Contemporary Autoethnography."
74. Discussions of these issues appear in, though are not limited to, the works of the following: Lynne D. Roberts, "Ethical Issues in Conducting Qualitative Research in Online Communities," *Qualitative Research in Psychology* 12, no. 3 (2015): 314–25; Cheryl Cooky, Jasmine R. Linabary, and Danielle J. Corple, "Navigating Big Data Dilemmas: Feminist Holistic Reflexivity in Social Media Research," *Big Data & Society* 5, no. 2 (2018): 1–12; Jennifer Germain, Jane Harris, Sean Mackay, and Clare Maxwell, "Why Should We Use Online Research Methods? Four Doctoral Health Student Perspectives," *Qualitative Health Research* 28, no. 10 (2018): 1650–57.
75. Some of those positions are represented by these works: Gunther Eysenbach and James E. Till, "Ethical Issues in Qualitative Research on Internet Communities," *BMJ* 323, no. 7321 (2001): 1103–5; Robert V. Kozinets, "The Field Behind the Screen: Using Netnography for Marketing Research in Online Communities," *Journal of Marketing Research* 39, no. 1 (2002): 61–72; Robert V. Kozinets, *Netnography: Ethnographic Research in the Age of the Internet* (Thousand Oaks, Calif.: Sage, 2010); Paul Reilly and Filippo Trevisan, "Researching Protest on Facebook: Developing an Ethical Stance for the Study of Northern Irish Flag Protest Pages," *Information, Communication & Society* 19, no. 3 (2016): 419–35; Barry Brown, Alexandra Weilenmann, Donald McMillan, and Airi Lampinen, "Five Provocations for Ethical HCI Research," in *Proceedings of the 2016 CHI Conference on Human Factors in Computing Systems* (2016): 852–63. 2016; Casey Fiesler and Nicholas Proferes, "'Participant' Perceptions of Twitter Research Ethics," *Social Media + Society* 4, no. 1 (2018): 1–14; Christian Pentzold, "'What Are These Researchers Doing in My Wikipedia?': Ethical Premises and Practical Judgment in Internet-Based Ethnography," *Ethics and Information Technology* 19, no. 2 (2017): 143–55; Charles Ess, *Digital Media Ethics* (Malden, Mass.: Polity, 2013); Michael Henderson, Nicola F. Johnson, and Glenn Auld, "Silences of Ethical Practice: Dilemmas for Researchers Using Social Media," *Educational Research and Evaluation* 19, no. 6 (2013): 546–60.
76. Elfriede Fürsich, "In Defense of Textual Analysis," *Journalism Studies* 10, no. 2 (2009): 241.
77. For examples of those critiques see Paul Du Gay, Stuart Hall, Linda Janes, Anders Koed Madsen, Hugh Mackay, and Keith Negus, *Doing Cultural Studies: The Story of the Sony Walkman* (Thousand Oaks,

Calif.: Sage, 2013); Greg Philo, "Can Discourse Analysis Successfully Explain the Content of Media and Journalistic Practice?," *Journalism Studies* 8, no. 2 (2007): 175–96.

78. Michelle Phillipov, "In Defense of Textual Analysis: Resisting Methodological Hegemony in Media and Cultural Studies," *Critical Studies in Media Communication* 30, no. 3 (2013): 210–11.
79. I am incredibly grateful to the anonymous reviewer who suggested this title for a coda. Thank you.

1. Mental Wellness by Smartphone App

1. The advertisement no longer is broadcasted, but it can be found on YouTube and in media coverage. See "iPhone 3g Commercial 'There's an App for That' 2009," February 4, 2009, https://www.youtube.com.
2. "Introducing Snap It™ By Lose It!," Lose It!, 2020, https://www.loseit.com/snapit/.
3. "Flo—Ovulation Calendar, Period Tracker, and Pregnancy App," Flo, 2020, https://flo.health/.
4. Michael V. Copeland, "New App Turns Your iPhone into a Mobile Urine Lab," *Wired,* February 26, 2013, https://www.wired.com.
5. "HAPI.com," HAPILABS, 2020, https://www.hapilabs.com.
6. Katrina Pascual, "Deodorant Manufacturer Nivea Launches Body Odor-Detecting App," *Tech Times* 26, 2016, https://www.techtimes.com/.
7. "Sleep Cycle: Sleep Tracker, Monitor & Alarm Clock," Sleep Cycle, June 22, 2020, https://www.sleepcycle.com/.
8. Stephen M. Schueller, Martha Neary, Kristen O'Loughlin, and Elizabeth C. Adkins, "Discovery of and Interest in Health Apps among Those with Mental Health Needs: Survey and Focus Group Study," *Journal of Medical Internet Research* 20, no. 6 (2018): e10141.
9. Stefan G. Hofmann, Anu Asnaani, Imke J. J. Vonk, Alice T. Sawyer, and Angela Fang, "The Efficacy of Cognitive Behavioral Therapy: A Review of Meta-Analyses," *Cognitive Therapy and Research* 36, no. 5 (2012): 427–40.
10. Christine Moberg, Andrea Niles, and Dale Beermann, "Guided Self-Help Works: Randomized Waitlist Controlled Trial of Pacifica, a Mobile App Integrating Cognitive Behavioral Therapy and Mindfulness for Stress, Anxiety, and Depression," *Journal of Medical Internet Research* 21, no. 6 (2019): e12556; Louise Champion, Marcos Economides, and Chris Chandler, "The Efficacy of a Brief App-Based Mindfulness Intervention on Psychosocial Outcomes in Healthy Adults: A Pilot Randomised Controlled Trial," *PloS One* 13, no. 12 (2018).

11. Kevin W. Chen, Christine C. Berger, Eric Manheimer, Darlene Forde, Jessica Magidson, Laya Dachman, and C. W. Lejuez, "Meditative Therapies for Reducing Anxiety: A Systematic Review and Meta-Analysis of Randomized Controlled Trials," *Depression and Anxiety* 29, no. 7 (2012): 545–62; Madhav Goyal, Sonal Singh, Erica M. S. Sibinga, Neda F. Gould, Anastasia Rowland-Seymour, Ritu Sharma, Zackary Berger, et al., "Meditation Programs for Psychological Stress and Well-Being: A Systematic Review and Meta-Analysis," *JAMA Internal Medicine* 174, no. 3 (2014): 357–68; Bassam Khoury, Tania Lecomte, Guillaume Fortin, Marjolaine Masse, Phillip Therien, Vanessa Bouchard, Marie-Andrée Chapleau, Karine Paquin, and Stefan G. Hofmann, "Mindfulness-Based Therapy: A Comprehensive Meta-Analysis," *Clinical Psychology Review* 33, no. 6 (2013): 763–71.
12. The FDA completed its revision to its policies about medical applications in 2019. For more information about those updates and prior policies, see "Policy for Device Software Functions and Mobile Medical Applications: Guidance for Industry and Food and Drug Administration Staff," Food and Drug Administration, September 27, 2019, https://www.fda.gov.
13. "App Evaluation Model," American Psychiatric Association, 2020, https://www.psychiatry.org.
14. "NHS Mental Health Apps Library to Increase Access to Psychological Therapies and Help to Improve Mental Health Outcomes," National Health Service, March 24, 2015, https://www.england.nhs.uk/.
15. Paul Wicks, and Emil Chiauzzi, "'Trust but Verify'—Five Approaches to Ensure Safe Medical Apps," *BMC Medicine* 13, no. 1 (2015): 1–5.
16. Eric Wicklund, "UK Tries Again with a Library of Certified Mobile Health Apps," *mHealth Intelligence,* April 21, 2017, https://mhealthintelligence.com.
17. Examples of research that has tried to show these applications do have beneficial outcomes include, but are not limited to, the following: Dror Ben-Zeev, Emily A. Scherer, Rui Wang, Haiyi Xie, and Andrew T. Campbell, "Next-Generation Psychiatric Assessment: Using Smartphone Sensors to Monitor Behavior and Mental Health," *Psychiatric Rehabilitation Journal* 38, no. 3 (2015): 218–26; John Torous, Patrick Staples, and Jukka-Pekka Onnela, "Realizing the Potential of Mobile Mental Health: New Methods for New Data in Psychiatry," *Current Psychiatry Reports* 17, no. 8 (2015): 61; Till Beiwinkel, Sally Kindermann, Andreas Maier, Christopher Kerl, Jörn Moock, Guido Barbian, and Wulf Rössler, "Using Smartphones to Monitor Bipolar Disorder Symptoms: A Pilot Study," *JMIR Mental Health* 3, no. 1 (2016): e2; Andreia Nunes, São Luís Castro, and Teresa Limpo,

"A Review of Mindfulness-Based Apps for Children," *Mindfulness* 11, no. 9 (2020): 2089–101.

18. "What Is Health 2.0?," Health 2.0, 2016, http://health2con.com/about.
19. Biographical information about Matthew Holt and Indu Sabaiya can be found on the Health 2.0 organization's website, http://health2con.com/about/our-team/.
20. "38th Annual J. P. Morgan Healthcare Conference," J. P. Morgan, 2020, https://www.jpmorgan.com.
21. "The Julia Morgan Ballroom," Julia Morgan Ballroom, 2017, https://juliamorganballroom.com.
22. The digital divide is discussed, analyzed, and critiqued across disciplines. For some notable examples of work on this topic see Benjamin M. Compaine, *The Digital Divide: Facing a Crisis or Creating a Myth?* (Cambridge, Mass.: MIT Press, 2001); Pippa Norris, *Digital Divide: Civic Engagement, Information Poverty, and the Internet Worldwide* (New York: Cambridge University Press, 2001).
23. "Our Story," Verily, 2020, https://verily.com.
24. There are different conceptualizations and definitions of "big data." For some examples see: Kirstie Ball, MariaLaura Di Domenico, and Daniel Nunan, "Big Data Surveillance and the Body-Subject," *Body & Society* 22, no. 2 (2016): 58–81; Gianluca Trifirò, Janet Sultana, and Andrew Bate, "From Big Data to Smart Data for Pharmacovigilance: The Role of Healthcare Databases and Other Emerging Sources," *Drug Safety* 41, no. 2 (2018): 143–49; Isitor Emmanuel and Clare Stanier, "Defining Big Data," *Proceedings of the International Conference on Big Data and Advanced Wireless Technologies* (2016): 1–6.
25. Fernando Iafrate, *From Big Data to Smart Data* (Hoboken, N.J.: John Wiley & Sons, 2015).
26. Examples of legal scholarship about privacy concerns include Michelle M. Christovich, "Why Should We Care What Fitbit Shares—A Proposed Statutory Solution to Protect Sensitive Personal Fitness Information," *Hastings Communications and Entertainment Law Journal* 38, no. 1 (2016): 91; Paige Papandrea, "Addressing the HIPAA-Potamus Sized Gap in Wearable Technology Regulation," *Minnesota Law Review* 104 (2019): 1095–132; Lori Andrews, "A New Privacy Paradigm in the Age of Apps," *Wake Forest Law Review* 53 (2018): 421–77.
27. Michael Bauer, Tasha Glenn, Scott Monteith, Rita Bauer, Peter C. Whybrow, and John Geddes, "Ethical Perspectives on Recommending Digital Technology for Patients with Mental Illness," *International Journal of Bipolar Disorders* 5, no. 1 (2017): 2.
28. Jonah Comstock, "Survey: One in Three People Tracks Health, Fitness with an App or Device," *Mobi Health News*, September 29, 2016, https://www.mobihealthnews.com/.

29. Digital phenotyping is a relatively new idea, but many find its possibilities exciting. For more discussion see Thomas R. Insel, "Digital Phenotyping: Technology for a New Science of Behavior," *JAMA*, 318, no. 13 (2017): 1215–16; Sachin H. Jain, Brian W. Powers, Jared B. Hawkins, and John S. Brownstein, "The Digital Phenotype," *Nature Biotechnology* 33, no. 5 (2015): 462.
30. For examples of this work see Sunghyun Yoon, Jai Kyoung Sim, and Young-Ho Cho, "A Flexible and Wearable Human Stress Monitoring Patch," *Scientific Reports* 6 (2016): 23468; Enrique Garcia-Ceja, Michael Riegler, Tine Nordgreen, Petter Jakobsen, Ketil J. Oedegaard, and Jim Tørresen, "Mental Health Monitoring with Multimodal Sensing and Machine Learning: A Survey," *Pervasive and Mobile Computing* 51 (2018): 1–26.
31. For examples see Rachel Metz, "The Smartphone App that Can Tell You're Depressed Before You Know It Yourself," *Technology Review,* October 15, 2018, https://www.technologyreview.com; Rafail-Evangelos Mastoras, Dimitrios Iakovakis, Stelios Hadjidimitriou, Vasileios Charisis, Seada Kassie, Taoufik Alsaadi, Ahsan Khandoker, and Leontios J. Hadjileontiadis, "Touchscreen Typing Pattern Analysis for Remote Detection of the Depressive Tendency," *Scientific Reports* 9, no. 1 (2019): 1–12; Nicholas D. Lane, Mashfiqui Mohammod, Mu Lin, Xiaochao Yang, Hong Lu, Shahid Ali, Afsaneh Doryab, Ethan Berke, Tanzeem Choudhury, and Andrew Campbell, "BeWell: A Smartphone Application to Monitor, Model and Promote Wellbeing," *5th International ICST Conference on Pervasive Computing Technologies for Healthcare* (2011): 23–26.
32. Adrian Aguilera and Frederick Muench, "There's an App for That: Information Technology Applications for Cognitive Behavioral Practitioners," *Behavior Therapist* 35, no. 4 (2012): 65–73.
33. Tim O'Reilly, "The World's 7 Most Powerful Data Scientists," *Forbes,* November 2, 2011, https://www.forbes.com/.
34. See some of those discussions and critiques from David Hunter and Nicholas Evans, "Facebook Emotional Contagion Experiment Controversy," *Research Ethics* 12, no.1 (2016): 2–3; Carl Elliott, "The Best-Selling, Billion-Dollar Pills Tested on Homeless People," *Medium,* July 28, 2014, https://medium.com; Carl Elliott, "The University of Minnesota's Medical Research Mess," *New York Times,* May 26, 2015, https://www.nytimes.com/.
35. This continues to be debated and contested, and opinions vary. See some positions represented in the following work: Gemma Stevens, Victoria L. O'Donnell, and Lynn Williams, "Public Domain or Private Data? Developing an Ethical Approach to Social Media Research in an Inter-Disciplinary Project," *Educational Research and Evaluation* 21,

no. 2 (2015): 154–67; Michael Zimmer, "'But the Data is Already Public': On the Ethics of Research in Facebook," *Ethics and Information Technology* 12, no. 4 (2010): 313–25; Matthew Zook, Solon Barocas, danah boyd, Kate Crawford, Emily Keller, Seeta Peña Gangadharan, Alyssa Goodman, et al., "Ten Simple Rules for Responsible Big Data Research," *PLOS Computational Biology* 13, no. 3 (2017): e1005399; Casey Fiesler and Nicholas Proferes, "'Participant' Perceptions of Twitter Research Ethics," *Social Media + Society* 4, no. 1 (2018): 1–14.

36. Sharath Chandra Guntuku, J. Russell Ramsay, Raina M. Merchant, and Lyle H. Ungar, "Language of ADHD in Adults on Social Media," *Journal of Attention Disorders* 23, no. 12 (2017): 1483.
37. Samantha Murphy, "Facebook Changes Its 'Move Fast and Break Things' Motto," *Mashable,* April 30, 2014, https://mashable.com.
38. In the introduction to this book I discussed medicalization and psychiatrization. See Nikolas Rose, "Disorders Without Borders? The Expanding Scope of Psychiatric Practice," *BioSocieties* 1, no. 4 (2006): 474; Peter Conrad, *The Medicalization of Society: On the Transformation of Human Conditions into Treatable Disorders* (Baltimore, Md.: Johns Hopkins University Press, 2007).
39. I believe he was referring to Siri, Apple's voice assistant. See "Siri Does More Than Ever. Even Before You Ask," Apple, 2020, https://www.apple.com.
40. Arlie Hochschild's research was some of the first to highlight emotional labor and management, and to point out that it is women who are largely called upon to have jobs that demand that work. See Arlie Hochschild, *The Managed Heart: Commercialization of Human Feeling* (Berkeley: University of California Press, 1983). Dominant trends within affect studies include scholarship on gendered labor and a longstanding interest, particularly within feminist media studies, with "affective registers" and women's "emotional labor." For examples of this scholarship see Sara Ahmed, "Not in the Mood," *New Formations* 82, no. 82 (2014): 13–28; Melissa Gregg, Gregory J. Seigworth, and Sara Ahmed, eds., *The Affect Theory Reader* (Durham, N.C.: Duke University Press, 2010); Imogen Tyler, Rebecca Coleman, and Debra Ferreday, "Methodological Fatigue and the Politics of the Affective Turn," *Feminist Media Studies* 8, no. 1 (2008): 85–99.
41. For more information on what it means to "access" healthcare, see Martin Gulliford, Jose Figueroa-Munoz, Myfanwy Morgan, David Hughes, Barry Gibson, Roger Beech, and Meryl Hudson, "What Does 'Access to Health Care' Mean?" *Journal of Health Services Research & Policy* 7, no. 3 (2002): 186–88.
42. See Simone Browne, "Digital Epidermalization: Race, Identity and Biometrics," *Critical Sociology* 36, no. 1 (2010): 131–50.

43. Quentin Hardy, "Looking for a Choice of Voice in AI Technology," *New York Times,* October 9, 2016, https://www.nytimes.com. Siri is one such application with a voice, but one that is also "white" sounding. See Taylor C. Moran, "Racial Technological Bias and the White, Feminine Voice of AI VAs," *Communication and Critical/Cultural Studies* (2020): 1–18.
44. Paul N. Edwards, "The Army and the Microworld: Computers and the Politics of Gender Identity," *Signs: Journal of Women in Culture and Society* 16, no. 1 (1990): 102.

2. Psychosurveillance

1. "A Facebook Algorithm That's Designed for Suicide Prevention," *NBC News,* January 18, 2018, www.nbcnews.com.
2. "A Facebook Algorithm That's Designed for Suicide Prevention," *NBC News.*
3. Emily Friedman, "Florida Teen Live-Streams His Suicide Online," *ABC News,* November 21, 2008, http://abcnews.go.com.
4. Friedman, "Florida Teen Live-Streams His Suicide Online."
5. Friso van Houdt and Willem Schinkel, "Crime, Citizenship and Community: Neoliberal Communitarian Images of Governmentality," *Sociological Review* 62, no. 1 (2014): 47.
6. Kenneth Cukier and Viktor Mayer-Schoenberger, "The Rise of Big Data: How It's Changing the Way We Think about the World," *Foreign Affairs* 92 (2013): 28–40.
7. While most attribute the idea of the panopticon to Jeremy Bentham, it was actually originally conceived of by his brother, Samuel Bentham. See Philip Steadman, "Samuel Bentham's Panopticon," *Journal of Bentham Studies* 14, no. 1 (2012): 1–30. Regardless, Jeremy Bentham was the one to publish about the panopticon in 1791. See Jeremy Bentham, *The Panopticon Writings,* ed. Miran Božovič (New York: Verso Books, 2011).
8. Ivan Manokha, "Surveillance, Panopticism, and Self-Discipline in the Digital Age," *Surveillance & Society* 16, no. 2 (2018): 222.
9. Michel Foucault, *Discipline and Punish: The Birth of the Prison,* trans. Alan Sheridan (New York: Vintage Books, 1977).
10. Hille Koskela, "'Cam Era'—The Contemporary Urban Panopticon," *Surveillance & Society* 1, no. 3 (2003): 292–313.
11. Examples of this scholarship include Manuela Farinosi, "Deconstructing Bentham's Panopticon: The New Metaphors of Surveillance in the Web 2.0 Environment," *TripleC: Communication, Capitalism & Critique* 9, no. 1 (2011): 62–67; Alberto Romele, Francesco Gallino, Camilla Emmenegger, and Daniele Gorgone, "Panopticism Is Not

Enough: Social Media as Technologies of Voluntary Servitude," *Surveillance & Society* 15, no. 2 (2017): 204–21.

12. See examples from Jean-François De Moya and Jessie Pallud, "From Panopticon to Heautopticon: A New Form of Surveillance Introduced by Quantified-Self Practices," *Information Systems Journal* (2020): 940–76; Katherine Hepworth, "A Panopticon on My Wrist: The Biopower of Big Data Visualization for Wearables," *Design and Culture* 11, no. 3 (2019): 323–44.
13. Mark Andrejevic, "The Discipline of Watching: Detection, Risk, and Lateral Surveillance," *Critical Studies in Media Communication* 23, no. 5 (2006): 397.
14. Andrejevic, "The Discipline of Watching," 393.
15. Examples include research from Tarleton Gillespie, *Custodians of the Internet: Platforms, Content Moderation, and the Hidden Decisions That Shape Social Media* (New Haven, Conn.: Yale University Press, 2018); Sarah T. Roberts, *Behind the Screen: Content Moderation in the Shadows of Social Media* (New Haven, Conn.: Yale University Press, 2019); Sarah T. Roberts, "Commercial Content Moderation: Digital Laborers' Dirty Work," in *The Intersectional Internet: Race, Sex, Class, and Culture Online,* ed. Safiya Noble and Brendesha M. Tynes (New York: Peter Lang, 2016), 147–60.
16. This received a significant amount of media attention. See Paige Leskin, "Mark Zuckerberg Calls Reports of Facebook Content Moderators Suffering PTSD after Watching Videos of People Dying 'A Little Overdramatic,'" *Business Insider,* October 1, 2019, https://www.businessinsider.com; Casey Newton, "Bodies in Seats," *The Verge,* June 19, 2019, https://www.theverge.com/; Terry Gross, "For Facebook Content Moderators, Traumatizing Material Is a Job Hazard," *Fresh Air,* July 1, 2019, https://www.npr.org.
17. Bobby Allyn, "In Settlement, Facebook to Pay $52 Million to Content Moderators with PTSD," *NPR,* May 12, 2020, https://www.npr.org.
18. Kate Crawford and Tarleton Gillespie, "What Is a Flag For? Social Media Reporting Tools and the Vocabulary of Complaint," *New Media & Society* 18, no. 3 (2016): 411.
19. Crawford and Gillespie, "What Is a Flag For?," 411.
20. Yasmin Ibrahim, "Facebook and the Napalm Girl: Reframing the Iconic as Pornographic," *Social Media + Society* 3, no. 4 (2017): 1–10.
21. For example, Instagram has removed images of breasts with mastectomy scars. See: Pippa Kent, "My Scars Aren't 'Sexual'—So Why Did Instagram Remove My Pictures?," *The Telegraph,* September 11, 2020, https://www.telegraph.co.uk.
22. Crawford and Gillespie, "What Is a Flag For?," 412.
23. "Support on Social Media," National Suicide Prevention Lifeline, 2020, https://suicidepreventionlifeline.org.

24. Alexis Kleinman, "Facebook Adds New Feature for Suicide Prevention," *Huffington Post*, February 25, 2015, http://www.huffingtonpost.com.
25. "About," Facebook Safety, 2020, https://www.facebook.com/.
26. Mark Zuckerberg, "Here's a Good Use of AI: Helping Prevent Suicide," Facebook, November 27, 2017, https://www.facebook.com.
27. Benjamin Goggin, "Inside Facebook's Suicide Algorithm: Here's How the Company Uses Artificial Intelligence to Predict Your Mental State from Your Posts," *Business Insider*, January 6, 2019, https://www.businessinsider.com.
28. Goggin, "Inside Facebook's Suicide Algorithm."
29. Natasha Singer, "In Screening for Suicide Risk, Facebook Takes on Tricky Public Health Role," *New York Times*, December 31, 2018, https://nytimes.com.
30. Some of the discussions about AI's usefulness in medicine can be found in the following works: Alex John London, "Artificial Intelligence and Black-Box Medical Decisions: Accuracy Versus Explainability," *Hastings Center Report* 49, no. 1 (2019): 15–21; Fei Wang, Rainu Kaushal, and Dhruv Khullar, "Should Health Care Demand Interpretable Artificial Intelligence or Accept "Black Box" Medicine?" *Annals of Internal Medicine* 172, no. 1 (2020): 59–60; W. Nicholson Price, "Regulating Black-Box Medicine," *Michigan Law Review* 116, no. 3 (2017): 421–74.
31. Drew Harwell, "Zuckerberg Says AI Will Solve Facebook's Problems, Mark Zuckerberg Says. Just Don't Ask How or When," *Washington Post*, April 12, 2018, https://www.washingtonpost.com.
32. When I was a graduate student, I asked a colleague to report a Facebook status post of mine as indicating intent to self-harm, purely for the purposes of research. I omitted a description of those events from this book because, to be frank, nothing really happened. I received a message from Facebook that was automated, letting me know that someone was concerned about my mental health, but that was the extent of the experiment. I have not, however, ever had a livestream reported upon. I no longer have a Facebook account and believe I got rid of it before the livestream function debuted. Therefore, for the description of processes related to livestreams being reported, I relied upon information presented in the following article: Megan Rose Dickey, "Facebook Brings Suicide Prevention Tools to Live and Messenger," *Tech Crunch*, March 1, 2017, https://techcrunch.com.
33. Nicolas Vega, "Facebook: We Can't Stop All Live-Stream Suicides," *New York Post*, October 25, 2017, https://nypost.com.
34. Vega, "Facebook."
35. Nick Hopkins, "Revealed: Facebook's Internal Rulebook on Sex, Terrorism and Violence," *The Guardian*, May 21, 2017, https://www.theguardian.com.

36. Nick Hopkins, "Facebook Will Let Users Livestream Self-Harm, Leaked Documents Show," *The Guardian*, May 21, 2017, https://www.theguardian.com.
37. David P. Phillips, "The Influence of Suggestion on Suicide: Substantive and Theoretical Implications of the Werther Effect," *American Sociological Review* 39, no. 3 (1974): 340–54.
38. For research on suicide contagion and social media, see Robert A. Fahey, Tetsuya Matsubayashi, and Michiko Ueda, "Tracking the Werther Effect on Social Media: Emotional Responses to Prominent Suicide Deaths on Twitter and Subsequent Increases in Suicide," *Social Science & Medicine* 219 (2018): 19–29; Lindsay Robertson, Keren Skegg, Marion Poore, Sheila Williams, and Barry Taylor, "An Adolescent Suicide Cluster and the Possible Role of Electronic Communication Technology," *Crisis* 33 (2012): 239–45; David D. Luxton, Jennifer D. June, and Jonathan M. Fairall, "Social Media and Suicide: A Public Health Perspective," *American Journal of Public Health* 102, no. S2 (2012): S195–S200.
39. "Company Info," Facebook, 2019, https://newsroom.fb.com.
40. John A. Naslund, Kelly A. Aschbrenner, Lisa Marsch, and Stephen Bartels, "The Future of Mental Health Care: Peer-to-Peer Support and Social Media," *Epidemiology and Psychiatric Sciences* 25, no. 2 (2016): 113–22; John A. Naslund, Stuart W. Grande, Kelly A. Aschbrenner, and Glyn Elwyn, "Naturally Occurring Peer Support through Social Media: The Experiences of Individuals with Severe Mental Illness Using YouTube," *PLOS one* 9, no. 10 (2014): e110171; Elizabeth Highton-Williamson, Stefan Priebe, and Domenico Giacco, "Online Social Networking in People with Psychosis: A Systematic Review," *International Journal of Social Psychiatry* 61, no. 1 (2015): 92–101.
41. "About 7 Cups," 7 Cups of Tea, 2020, https://www.7cups.com.
42. "Become an Online Volunteer Listener," 7 Cups of Tea, 2020, https://www.7cups.com.
43. This research is cited on the 7 Cups of Tea website: Amit Baumel, "Online Emotional Support Delivered by Trained Volunteers: Users' Satisfaction and Their Perception of the Service Compared to Psychotherapy," *Journal of Mental Health* 24, no. 5 (2015): 313–20; Amit Baumel, Amanda Tinkelman, Nandita Mathur, and John M. Kane, "Digital Peer-Support Platform (7Cups) as an Adjunct Treatment for Women with Postpartum Depression: Feasibility, Acceptability, and Preliminary Efficacy Study," *JMIR mHealth and uHealth* 6, no. 2 (2018): e38; Amit Baumel, Christoph U. Correll, and Michael Birnbaum, "Adaptation of a Peer Based Online Emotional Support Program as an Adjunct to Treatment for People with Schizophrenia-Spectrum Disorders," *Internet Interventions* 4 (2016): 35–42; Amit Baumel and Stephen M. Schueller, "Adjusting an Available Online Peer Support Platform in a Program to Supplement

the Treatment of Perinatal Depression and Anxiety," *JMIR Mental Health* 3, no. 1 (2016): e11.

44. "Listener Training," 7 Cups of Tea, 2018, https://www.7cups.com.
45. Otto Wahl, "Stop the Presses: Journalistic Treatment of Mental Illness," in *Cultural Sutures: Medicine and Media,* ed. Lester D. Friedman (Durham, N.C.: Duke University Press, 2004), 55.
46. For examples of research suggesting the positive effects of destigmatizing campaigns, see Amalia Thornicroft, Robert Goulden, Guy Shefer, Danielle Rhydderch, Diana Rose, Paul Williams, Graham Thornicroft, and Claire Henderson, "Newspaper Coverage of Mental Illness in England 2008–2011," *British Journal of Psychiatry* 202, no. s55 (2013): s64–s69; Heather Stuart, "Stigma and the Daily News: Evaluation of a Newspaper Intervention," *Canadian Journal of Psychiatry* 48, no. 10 (2003): 651–56; Patrick Corrigan, and Betsy Gelb, "Three Programs that Use Mass Approaches to Challenge the Stigma of Mental Illness," *Psychiatric Services* 57, no. 3 (2006): 393–98.
47. Nikolas Rose, *Inventing Our Selves: Psychology, Power, and Personhood* (New York: Cambridge University Press, 1998), vii.
48. At the very least, this is what I told myself.
49. Alice Gregory, "R U There?" *New Yorker,* February 2, 2015, https://www.newyorker.com.
50. "Crisis Trends," Crisis Text Line, 2020, https://crisistrends.org.
51. "Become a Crisis Counselor," Crisis Text Line, 2020, https://www.crisistextline.org.
52. There are a number of blog posts wherein volunteers share their positive feelings about being Crisis Counselors. Two such posts on this topic are titled "Saving Lives Before You Sleep" and "I Was Stuck in a Rut. Becoming a Crisis Counselor Gave Me a New Spark." The Crisis Text Line *Everyday Empathy* blog can be found at https://www.crisistextline.org/everyday-empathy.
53. In 2019 Crisis Text Line won a Skoll World Forum award. See Nina Sachdev, "Meet Crisis Text Line, One of the Winners of This Year's Skoll World Forum on Social Entrepreneurship Awards," Media Impact Funders, April 5, 2019, https://mediaimpactfunders.org.
54. Nancy Lublin, "5 Things Crisis Text Line Learned by Going Global in 2018," Crisis Text Line, 2018, https://www.crisistextline.org.
55. Kylie Jarrett, "The Relevance of 'Women's Work': Social Reproduction and Immaterial Labor in Digital Media," *Television & New Media* 15, no. 1 (2014): 14.

3. Chatbots and Therapeutic AI

1. Adrienne Mayor, *Gods and Robots: Myths, Machines, and Ancient Dreams of Technology* (Princeton, N.J.: Princeton University Press, 2020), 1.

2. Mayor, *Gods and Robots*, 1.
3. Libby Plummer, "This Is How Netflix's Top-Secret Recommendation System Works," *Wired*, August 22, 2017, https://www.wired.co.uk.
4. Kevin Kelleher, "How Artificial Intelligence Is Quietly Changing How You Shop Online," *Time*, March 1, 2017, https://time.com.
5. Daniel Martin, "Cortana vs. Siri vs. Google Assistant vs. Alexa," *Digital Trends*, September 23, 2020, https://www.digitaltrends.com.
6. Lara Zarum, "Some Viewers Think Netflix Is Targeting Them by Race. Here's What to Know," *New York Times*, October 23, 2018, https://www.nytimes.com.
7. Ray Fisman and Michael Luca, "Fixing Discrimination in Online Marketplaces," *Harvard Business Review*, December 2016, https://hbr.org.
8. This has been noticed by academics and journalists. See Cade Metz, "There Is a Racial Divide in Speech-Recognition Systems, Researchers Say," *New York Times*, March 23, 2020, https://www.nytimes.com; Allison Koenecke, Andrew Nam, Emily Lake, Joe Nudell, Minnie Quartey, Zion Mengesha, Connor Toups, John R. Rickford, Dan Jurafsky, and Sharad Goel, "Racial Disparities in Automated Speech Recognition," *Proceedings of the National Academy of Sciences* 117, no. 14 (2020): 7684–89.
9. For examples of popular discourse positioning chatbots as solutions to the mental healthcare crisis, see Esther Shein, "82% of People Believe Robots Can Support Their Mental Health Better than Humans," *Tech Republic*, October 7, 2020, https://www.techrepublic.com; Jonathan Burton, "Would You Tell Your Innermost Secrets to Alexa? How AI Therapists Could Save You Time and Money on Mental Health Care," *Market Watch*, February 22, 2020, https://www.marketwatch.com; Jamie Ducharme, "Artificial Intelligence Could Help Solve America's Impending Mental Health Crisis," *Time*, November 20, 2019, https://time.com.
10. Chukwuemeka Afigbo (@nke_ise), 2017, "If you have ever had a problem grasping the importance of diversity in tech and its impact on society, watch this video," Twitter, August 16, 2017, 5:45 a.m. https://twitter.com/nke_ise/status/897756900753891328.
11. Tom Hale, "This Video of a Racist Soap Dispenser Reveals a Much, Much Bigger Problem," *IFL Science*, August 18, 2017, https://www.iflscience.com.
12. Sage Lazzaro, "Is This Soap Dispenser Racist?," *Daily Mail*, August 17, 2017, https://www.dailymail.co.uk; Sidney Fussell, "Why Can't This Soap Dispenser Identify Dark Skin?," *Gizmodo*, August 17, 2017, https://gizmodo.com.
13. This is not the position taken by the author of the cited article, but is described clearly by him: Mark Maguire, "Biopower, Racialization and New Security Technology," *Social Identities* 18, no. 5 (2012): 594.

14. Simone Browne, “Digital Epidermalization: Race, Identity and Biometrics,” *Critical Sociology* 36, no. 1 (2010): 131–50.
15. Aja Romano, “Coronavirus Memes Let Us See Internet Humor Evolving Overnight,” *Vox,* March 23, 2020, https://www.vox.com; “How to Protect Yourself and Others,” *Centers for Disease Control,* April 13, 2020, http://www.cdc.gov.
16. Monica Brown, “Don’t Be the “Fifth Guy”: Risk, Responsibility, and the Rhetoric of Handwashing Campaigns,” *Journal of Medical Humanities* 40, no. 2 (2019): 212.
17. For one example of such a definition, see Jessen Havill, *Discovering Computer Science: Interdisciplinary Problems, Principles, and Python Programming* (Cleveland, Ohio: CRC Press, 2020), 7.
18. Ethem Alpaydin, *Introduction to Machine Learning* (Cambridge, Mass.: MIT Press, 2020), 3.
19. Yann LeCun, Yoshua Bengio, and Geoffrey Hinton, “Deep Learning,” *Nature* 521, no. 7553 (2015): 436–44.
20. Nick Seaver, “Knowing Algorithms,” in *A Field Guide for Science & Technology Studies,* ed. Janet Vertesi and David Ribes (Princeton, N.J.: Princeton University Press, 2019), 419.
21. Nils Johan Nilsson, *Artificial Intelligence: A New Synthesis* (San Francisco, Calif.: Morgan Kaufmann, 1998).
22. Alan M. Turing, “Computing Machinery and Intelligence,” *Mind* 59, no. 236 (1950): 433–60.
23. Paul Hsieh, “AI in Medicine: Rise of the Machines,” *Forbes,* April 30, 2017, https://www.forbes.com.
24. This perspective is not that humans will become obsolete, but rather that their abilities will be extended by AI. See Irene Y. Chen, Peter Szolovits, and Marzyeh Ghassemi, “Can AI Help Reduce Disparities in General Medical and Mental Health Care?” *AMA Journal of Ethics* 21, no. 2 (2019): 167–79.
25. Vivek Kaul, Sarah Enslin, and Seth A. Gross, “The History of Artificial Intelligence in Medicine,” *Gastrointestinal Endoscopy* 92, no. 4 (2020): 807–12.
26. Megan Garcia, “Racist in the Machine: The Disturbing Implications of Algorithmic Bias,” *World Policy Journal* 33, no. 4 (2016): 112.
27. Ziad Obermeyer, Brian Powers, Christine Vogeli, and Sendhil Mullainathan, “Dissecting Racial Bias in an Algorithm Used to Manage the Health of Populations,” *Science* 366, no. 6464 (2019): 447–53.
28. Ruha Benjamin, “Assessing Risk, Automating Racism,” *Science* 366, no. 6464 (2019): 421.
29. Obermeyer, Powers, Vogeli, and Mullainathan, “Dissecting Racial Bias,” 453.
30. Joseph Weizenbaum, “ELIZA—A Computer Program for the Study of Natural Language Communication Between Man and Machine,” *Communications of the ACM* 9, no. 1 (1966): 36–45; Rafael A.

Calvo, David N. Milne, M. Sazzad Hussain, and Helen Christensen, "Natural Language Processing in Mental Health Applications Using Non-Clinical Texts," *Natural Language Engineering* 23, no. 5 (2017): 649–85.

31. Weizenbaum, "ELIZA," 36–37.
32. Joseph Weizenbaum, *Computer Power and Human Reason: From Judgment to Calculation* (New York: W. H. Freeman, 1976).
33. Alaa A. Abd-alrazaq, Mohannad Alajlani, Ali Abdallah Alalwan, Bridgette M. Bewick, Peter Gardner, and Mowafa Househ, "An Overview of the Features of Chatbots in Mental Health: A Scoping Review," *International Journal of Medical Informatics* (2019): 2.
34. Simon Provoost, Ho Ming Lau, Jeroen Ruwaard, and Heleen Riper, "Embodied Conversational Agents in Clinical Psychology: A Scoping Review," *Journal of Medical Internet Research* 19, no. 5 (2017): e151.
35. Provoost, Lau, Ruwaard, and Riper, "Embodied Conversational Agents." See also Mary Bates, "Health Care Chatbots Are Here to Help," *IEEE Pulse* 10, no. 3 (2019): 12–14.
36. Brian J. Fogg, *Persuasive Technology: Using Computers to Change What We Think and Do* (New York: Morgan Kaufmann, 2003), 1.
37. Yang-Wai Chow, Willy Susilo, James G. Phillips, Joonsang Baek, and Elena Vlahu-Gjorgievska, "Video Games and Virtual Reality as Persuasive Technologies for Health Care: An Overview," *Journal of Wireless Mobile Networks, Ubiquitous Computing, and Dependable Applications* 8, no. 3 (2017): 18–35.
38. Julie B. Wang, Lisa A. Cadmus-Bertram, Loki Natarajan, Martha M. White, Hala Madanat, Jeanne F. Nichols, Guadalupe X. Ayala, and John P. Pierce, "Wearable Sensor/Device (Fitbit One) and SMS Text-Messaging Prompts to Increase Physical Activity in Overweight and Obese Adults: A Randomized Controlled Trial," *Telemedicine and e-Health* 21, no. 10 (2015): 782–92.
39. Jaap Ham, Raymond H. Cuijpers, and John-John Cabibihan, "Combining Robotic Persuasive Strategies: The Persuasive Power of a Storytelling Robot That Uses Gazing and Gestures," *International Journal of Social Robotics* 7, no. 4 (2015): 479–87.
40. Simona D'Oca, Stefano P. Corgnati, and Tiziana Buso, "Smart Meters and Energy Savings in Italy: Determining the Effectiveness of Persuasive Communication in Dwellings," *Energy Research & Social Science* 3 (2014): 131–42.
41. Oladapo Oyebode and Rita Orji, "Deconstructing Persuasive Strategies in Mental Health Apps Based on User Reviews Using Natural Language Processing," *CEUR International Workshop on Behavior Change Support Systems* (2020); Felwah Alqahtani, Ghazayil Al Khalifah, Oladapo Oyebode, and Rita Orji, "Apps for Mental Health: An Evaluation of Behavior Change Strategies and Recommenda-

tions for Future Development," *Frontiers in Artificial Intelligence* 2, no. 30 (2019).

42. "FAQ," Woebot, 2017, https://woebot.io.
43. For examples of scholarship on this topic see Clifford Nass and Youngme Moon, "Machines and Mindlessness: Social Responses to Computers," *Journal of Social Issues* 56, no. 1 (2000): 81–103; Li Gong, "How Social Is Social Responses to Computers? The Function of the Degree of Anthropomorphism in Computer Representations," *Computers in Human Behavior* 24, no. 4 (2008): 1494–509; Li Gong and Clifford Nass, "When a Talking-Face Computer Agent Is Half-Human and Half-Humanoid: Human Identity and Consistency Preference," *Human Communication Research* 33, no. 2 (2007): 163–93; Youjeong Kim and S. Shyam Sundar, "Anthropomorphism of Computers: Is It Mindful or Mindless?," *Computers in Human Behavior* 28, no. 1 (2012): 241–50.
44. Chris Fullwood, Sally Quinn, Linda K. Kaye, and Charlotte Redding, "My Virtual Friend: A Qualitative Analysis of the Attitudes and Experiences of Smartphone Users: Implications for Smartphone Attachment," *Computers in Human Behavior* 75 (2017): 347–55.
45. Gisli Thorsteinsson and Tom Page, "User Attachment to Smartphones and Design Guidelines," *International Journal of Mobile Learning and Organisation* 8, no. 3–4 (2014): 201–15.
46. Kathleen Kara Fitzpatrick, Alison Darcy, and Molly Vierhile, "Delivering Cognitive Behavior Therapy to Young Adults with Symptoms of Depression and Anxiety Using a Fully Automated Conversational Agent (Woebot): A Randomized Controlled Trial," *JMIR Mental Health* 4, no. 2 (2017): e20.
47. Fitzpatrick, Darcy, and Vierhile, "Delivering Cognitive Behavior Therapy."
48. Leslie J. Hinyard and Matthew W. Kreuter, "Using Narrative Communication as a Tool for Health Behavior Change: A Conceptual, Theoretical, and Empirical Overview," *Health Education & Behavior* 34, no. 5 (2007): 777–92; Fuyuan Shen, Vivian C. Sheer, and Ruobing Li, "Impact of Narratives on Persuasion in Health Communication: A Meta-Analysis," *Journal of Advertising* 44, no. 2 (2015): 105–13.
49. An emoji is "a graphic symbol, ideogram, that represents not only facial expressions, but also concepts and ideas, such as celebration, weather, vehicles and buildings, food and drink, animals and plants, or emotions, feelings, and activities." This definition is from Petra Kralj Novak, Jasmina Smailović, Borut Sluban, and Igor Mozetič, "Sentiment of Emojis," *PloS One* 10, no. 12 (2015): e0144296.
50. Even I am sometimes confused by what emojis mean. Adding to the confusion, the same emoji might be used by different people for

different reasons. See research on this from Vikas N. O'Reilly-Shah, Grant C. Lynde, and Craig S. Jabaley, "Is It Time to Start Using the Emoji in Biomedical Literature?," *BMJ* 363 (2018): 1–3.

51. Jessica Fitts Willoughby and Shuang Liu, "Do Pictures Help Tell the Story? An Experimental Test of Narrative and Emojis in a Health Text Message Intervention," *Computers in Human Behavior* 79 (2018): 75–82.
52. Fitzpatrick, Darcy, and Vierhile, "Delivering Cognitive Behavior Therapy," e19.
53. Megan Molteni, "The Chatbot Therapist Will See You Now," *Wired,* June 7, 2017, https://www.wired.com.
54. Erin Brodwin, "A Stanford Researcher Is Pioneering a Dramatic Shift in How We Treat Depression—And You Can Try Her New Tool Right Now," *Business Insider,* January 25, 2018, http://www.business insider.com.
55. Marie Boran, "Woebot Is There to Listen and Help Users Track Their Mood," *Irish Times,* February 8, 2018, https://www.irishtimes.com.
56. "Mobile Fact Sheet," Pew Research Center, June 12, 2019, https://www .pewinternet.org.
57. Shameen Alauddin, "Touchkin's Bot to Keep Tab on Your Mental Health," *Business Standard,* August 13, 2017, https://www.business -standard.com.
58. "Wysa," Wysa, 2020, https://www.wysa.io.
59. Eric Wallach, "An Interview with Jo Aggarwal, Co-Inventor of Wysa," *The Politic,* March 28, 2018, http://thepolitic.org.
60. Although I do not find this acronym to be entirely inclusive, it is what the Wysa program uses.
61. Aurea Falco and Sanjana Gandhi, "The Rainbow Business," *Eidos* 9, no. 1 (2019): 104–7.
62. Wallach, "An Interview with Jo Aggarwal."
63. Wallach, "An Interview with Jo Aggarwal."
64. Research demonstrates that multiple aspects of identity should be taken into account for CBT to be most effective. These include (but are not limited to) a person's gender identity, race, and socioeconomic status. See Liliane C. Windsor, Alexis Jemal, and Edward J. Alessi, "Cognitive Behavioral Therapy: A Meta-Analysis of Race and Substance Use Outcomes," *Cultural Diversity and Ethnic Minority Psychology* 21, no. 2 (2015): 300; Kristin Lester, Caroline Artz, Patricia A. Resick, and Yinong Young-Xu, "Impact of Race on Early Treatment Termination and Outcomes in Posttraumatic Stress Disorder Treatment," *Journal of Consulting and Clinical Psychology* 78, no. 4 (2010): 480–89; Ashley Austin and Shelley L. Craig, "Transgender Affirmative Cognitive Behavioral Therapy: Clinical Considerations and Applications," *Professional Psychology: Research and Practice* 46,

no. 1 (2015): 21–29; Saeromi Kim and Esteban Cardemil, "Effective Psychotherapy with Low-Income Clients: The Importance of Attending to Social Class," *Journal of Contemporary Psychotherapy* 42, no. 1 (2012): 27–35.

65. For examples see Ethan Watters, *Crazy Like Us: The Globalization of the American Psyche* (New York: Simon and Schuster, 2010); Gavin Miller, "Is the Agenda for Global Mental Health a Form of Cultural Imperialism?," *Medical Humanities* 40, no. 2 (2014): 131–34; Kenneth J. Gergen, Aydan Gulerce, Andrew Lock, and Girishwar Misra, "Psychological Science in Cultural Context," *American Psychologist* 51, no. 5 (1996): 496–503.
66. Research suggests that errors in texts lead to negative perceptions of those texts' authors, whether they are text messages or otherwise. See Kenneth J. Houghton, Sri Siddhi N. Upadhyay, and Celia M. Klin, "Punctuation in Text Messages May Convey Abruptness. Period," *Computers in Human Behavior* 80 (2018): 112–21; Adam C. Johnson, Joshua Wilson, and Rod D. Roscoe, "College Student Perceptions of Writing Errors, Text Quality, and Author Characteristics," *Assessing Writing* 34 (2017): 72–87; Julie E. Boland and Robin Queen, "If You're House Is Still Available, Send Me an Email: Personality Influences Reactions to Written Errors in Email Messages," *PloS One* 11, no. 3 (2016): e0149885.
67. Khari Johnson, "The Mental Health Tracker Joy Wants to Get More People Professional Help," *Venture Beat,* July 19, 2016, https://venturebeat.com.
68. Suzanne Bearne, "Meet the 'Doctors' Who Will Talk to You Whenever You Like," *BBC,* July 18, 2017, https://www.bbc.com; Nadhi Singh, "Are You Depressed? Talk to These Chatbots," *Entrepreneur,* June 9, 2017, https://www.entrepreneur.com.
69. "Help Center," Hello Joy, 2017, http://www.hellojoy.com.
70. "Help Center," Hello Joy.
71. Torin Monahan, "Algorithmic Fetishism," *Surveillance & Society* 16, no. 1 (2018): 2.
72. My use of the phrase "discriminatory design" should be attributed to Ruha Benjamin, whose scholarship has explored various iterations of discriminatory design for years. See "Benjamin Delves into 'Discriminatory Design' in Medical, Scientific Research," Princeton University, March 9, 2015, https://www.princeton.edu.
73. Monahan, "Algorithmic Fetishism," 2.
74. This is well established by research. See examples in scholarship from Liliane C. Windsor, Alexis Jemal, and Edward J. Alessi, "Cognitive Behavioral Therapy: A Meta-Analysis of Race and Substance Use Outcomes," *Cultural Diversity and Ethnic Minority Psychology* 21, no. 2 (2015): 300; Kristin Lester, Caroline Artz, Patricia A.

Resick, and Yinong Young-Xu, "Impact of Race on Early Treatment Termination and Outcomes in Posttraumatic Stress Disorder Treatment," *Journal of Consulting and Clinical Psychology* 78, no. 4 (2010): 480–89; Julia S. Seng, William D. Lopez, Mickey Sperlich, Lydia Hamama, and Caroline D. Reed Meldrum, "Marginalized Identities, Discrimination Burden, and Mental Health: Empirical Exploration of an Interpersonal-Level Approach to Modeling Intersectionality," *Social Science & Medicine* 75, no. 12 (2012): 2437–45; Kira Hudson Banks and Laura P. Kohn-Wood, "Gender, Ethnicity and Depression: Intersectionality in Mental Health Research with African American Women," *African American Research Perspectives* 6 (2002): 174–84; Edna A. Viruell-Fuentes, Patricia Y. Miranda, and Sawsan Abdulrahim, "More Than Culture: Structural Racism, Intersectionality Theory, and Immigrant Health," *Social Science & Medicine* 75, no. 12 (2012): 2099–106.

75. Mark Marino, "The Racial Formation of Chatbots," *CLCWeb: Comparative Literature and Culture* 16, no. 5 (2014): 2.
76. Marino, "The Racial Formation of Chatbots," 5.
77. "Internet/Broadband Fact Sheet," Pew Research Center, June 12, 2019, https://www.pewresearch.org.
78. Felicity de Zulueta, *From Pain to Violence—The Traumatic Roots of Destructiveness.* (London: Whurr, 1993); Farhad Dalal, "Racism: Processes of Detachment, Dehumanization, and Hatred," *Psychoanalytic Quarterly* 75, no. 1 (2006): 131–61.

4. Telemental Healthcare

1. This advertisement was uploaded to YouTube on August 29, 2012, but has since been taken down. However, the organization that uploaded it, Insight Telepsychiatry, still maintains a YouTube channel. The ad can still be viewed by utilizing the Wayback Machine: https://web.archive.org/web/20200505014226if_/https://www.youtube.com/watch?v=Dk9yMgqZa4Y.
2. "Telehealth: Defining 21st Century Care," American Telemedicine Association, 2020, https://www.americantelemed.org.
3. Bonnie Kaplan and Sergio Litewka, "Ethical Challenges of Telemedicine and Telehealth," *Cambridge Quarterly of Healthcare Ethics* 17 (2008): 401–16.
4. Jonathan D. Neufeld, Charles R. Doarn, and Reem Aly, "State Policies Influence Medicare Telemedicine Utilization," *Telemedicine and e-Health* 22, no. 1 (2016): 70–74; Anca M. Grecu and Ghanshyam Sharma, "The Effect of Telehealth Insurance Mandates on Health-Care Utilization and Outcomes," *Applied Economics* 51, no. 56 (2019): 5972–85.

5. "House Passes Guidelines on Teledentistry," American Dental Association, December 7, 2015, https://www.ada.org.
6. Jonathan J. Lee and Joseph C. English, "Teledermatology: A Review and Update," *American Journal of Clinical Dermatology* 19, no. 2 (2018): 253–60.
7. Andrea L. Greiner, "Telemedicine Applications in Obstetrics and Gynecology," *Clinical Obstetrics and Gynecology* 60, no. 4 (2017): 853–66.
8. Kate Cavanagh and Abigail Millings, "(Inter)personal Computing: The Role of the Therapeutic Relationship in E-Mental Health," *Journal of Contemporary Psychotherapy* 43, no. 4 (2013): 197–206; Heleen Riper, Gerhard Andersson, Helen Christensen, Pim Cuijpers, Alfred Lange, and Gunther Eysenbach, "Theme Issue on E-Mental Health: A Growing Field in Internet Research," *Journal of Medical Internet Research* 12, no. 5 (2010): e74.
9. Monique Manhal-Baugus, "E-therapy: Practical, Ethical, and Legal Issues," *CyberPsychology & Behavior* 4, no. 5 (2001): 551–63.
10. Adriana S. Miu, Hoa T. Vo, Jayme M. Palka, Christopher R. Glowacki, and Reed J. Robinson, "Teletherapy with Serious Mental Illness Populations During COVID-19: Telehealth Conversion and Engagement," *Counselling Psychology Quarterly* (2020): 1–18.
11. The term *telepsychiatry,* like *psychiatry,* specifically refers to care provided by persons with medical degrees. Telepsychiatrists, like psychiatrists, are therefore able to prescribe medications, which makes them distinct from therapists and psychologists. Sometimes, however, even the term *telepsychiatry* is used interchangeably with terms for mental healthcare provided at a distance. See Peter Yellowlees, Steven Richard Chan, and Michelle Burke Parish, "The Hybrid Doctor–Patient Relationship in the Age of Technology–Telepsychiatry Consultations and the Use of Virtual Space," *International Review of Psychiatry* 27, no. 6 (2015): 476–89.
12. Susan Simpson, Lisa K. Richardson, and Nadine Pelling, "Introduction to the Special Issue 'Telepsychology: Research and Practice,'" *Australian Psychologist* 50, no. 4 (2015): 249–51.
13. Donald M. Hilty, Daphne C. Ferrer, Michelle Burke Parish, Barb Johnston, Edward J. Callahan, and Peter M. Yellowlees, "The Effectiveness of Telemental Health: A 2013 Review," *Telemedicine and E-Health* 19, no. 6 (2013): 444–54.
14. Joint Task Force for the Development of Telepsychology Guidelines for Psychologists, "Guidelines for the Practice of Telepsychology," *American Psychologist* 68, no. 9 (2013): 792.
15. "Learn About Mental Health," Centers for Disease Control, 2018, https://www.cdc.gov.
16. "Mental Health Disparities: Diverse Populations," American Psychiatric Association, 2017, https://www.psychiatry.org; "Mental Illness,"

National Institute of Mental Health, 2019, https://www.nimh.nih.gov.

17. "Racial and Ethnic Disparities in Men's Use of Mental Health Treatments," Centers for Disease Control, 2015, https://www.cdc.gov.
18. Tahirah Abdullah and Tamara L. Brown, "Mental Illness Stigma and Ethnocultural Beliefs, Values, and Norms: An Integrative Review," *Clinical Psychology Review* 31, no. 6 (2011): 934–48; E. Jane Costello, Scott N. Compton, Gordon Keeler, and Adrian Angold, "Relationships Between Poverty and Psychopathology: A Natural Experiment," *JAMA* 290, no. 15 (2003): 2023–29; Eris F. Perese, "Stigma, Poverty, and Victimization: Roadblocks to Recovery for Individuals with Severe Mental Illness," *Journal of the American Psychiatric Nurses Association* 13, no. 5 (2007): 285–95; Erum Nadeem, Jane M. Lange, Dawn Edge, Marie Fongwa, Tom Belin, and Jeanne Miranda, "Does Stigma Keep Poor Young Immigrant and US-Born Black and Latina Women from Seeking Mental Health Care?," *Psychiatric Services* 58, no. 12 (2007): 1547–54.
19. Heather Kugelmass, "'Sorry, I'm Not Accepting New Patients': An Audit Study of Access to Mental Health Care," *Journal of Health and Social Behavior* 57, no. 2 (2016): 168–83.
20. "About Us," American Telemedicine Association, 2020, https://www.americantelemed.org.
21. "Policy," American Telemedicine Association, 2020, https://www.americantelemed.org.
22. Martin Gulliford, Jose Figueroa-Munoz, Myfanwy Morgan, David Hughes, Barry Gibson, Roger Beech, and Meryl Hudson, "What Does 'Access to Health Care' Mean?" *Journal of Health Services Research & Policy* 7, no. 3 (2002): 186–88.
23. April Dembosky, "Frustrated You Can't Find a Therapist? They're Frustrated, Too," *NPR*, July 14, 2016, www.npr.org.
24. Mujtaba Ahsan, "Entrepreneurship and Ethics in the Sharing Economy: A Critical Perspective," *Journal of Business Ethics* 161, no. 1 (2020): 19–33.
25. Jonathan V. Hall and Alan B. Krueger, "An Analysis of the Labor Market for Uber's Driver-Partners in the United States," *ILR Review* 71, no. 3 (2018): 705–32; Alex Rosenblat, *Uberland: How Algorithms Are Rewriting the Rules of Work* (Berkeley: University of California Press, 2018).
26. Ahsan, "Entrepreneurship and Ethics."
27. "Counselor Jobs," Better Help, 2020, https://www.betterhelp.com.
28. Cat Ferguson, "Breakdown," *The Verge*, (December 19, 2016, https://www.theverge.com.
29. Kylie Jarrett, "The Relevance of 'Women's Work' Social Reproduction and Immaterial Labor in Digital Media," *Television & New Media* 15, no. 1 (2014): 14–29.

30. Valerio De Stefano, "The Rise of the Just-in-Time Workforce: On-Demand Work, Crowdwork, and Labor Protection in the Gig-Economy," *Comparative. Labor Law & Policy Journal* 37 (2015): 471.
31. Gulliford, Figueroa-Munoz, Morgan, Hughes, Gibson, Beech, and Hudson, "What Does 'Access to Health Care' Mean?"

5. The Future of Mental Health Technologies

1. This is a pseudonym.
2. Simone Browne, "Digital Epidermalization: Race, Identity and Biometrics," *Critical Sociology* 36, no. 1 (2010): 131–50.
3. "Mental Health Disparities: Diverse Populations," American Psychiatric Association, 2017, https://www.psychiatry.org; "Mental Illness," National Institute of Mental Health, 2019, https://www.nimh.nih.gov/; "Racial and Ethnic Disparities in Men's Use of Mental Health Treatments," Centers for Disease Control, 2015, https://www.cdc.gov.
4. "Remarks by President Trump on the Mass Shootings in Texas and Ohio," The White House, August 5, 2019, https://www.whitehouse.gov.
5. Samuel C. Florman, *Blaming Technology: The Irrational Search for Scapegoats* (New York: Macmillan, 1981); Alice E. Marwick, "To Catch A Predator? The MySpace Moral Panic," *First Monday* 13, no. 6 (2008): https://firstmonday.org; Chris Ingraham and Joshua Reeves, "New Media, New Panics," *Critical Studies in Media Communication* 33, no. 5 (2016): 455–67.
6. William Wan, "White House Weighs Controversial Plan on Mental Illness and Mass Shootings," *Washington Post,* September 9, 2019, https://www.washingtonpost.com.
7. Paul Cobler, "After Santa Fe Shooting, Gov. Greg Abbott Wants to Put More Counselors in Schools. Educators Say That's Not Enough," *Texas Tribune,* June 12, 2018, https://www.texastribune.org; Bailey Gallion, "School Shootings: Mental Health Symptoms Parents Can Watch Out For," *Dayton Daily News,* May 24, 2018, https://www.daytondailynews.com; Louis Nelson, "Trump Says He'll Visit Florida, Emphasize Mental Health After School Shooting," *Politico,* February 15, 2018, https://www.politico.com; Daniel Victor, "School Shootings Have Already Killed Dozens in 2018," *New York Times,* May 18, 2018, https://www.nytimes.com.
8. See examples from Dana Lee Baker, *The Politics of Neurodiversity: Why Public Policy Matters* (Boulder, Colo.: Lynne Rienner, 2011); Katherine Runswick-Cole, "'Us' and 'Them': The Limits and Possibilities of a 'Politics of Neurodiversity' in Neoliberal Times," *Disability & Society* 29, no. 7 (2014): 1117–29.

COVID Coda

1. Emily A. Vogels, Andrew Perrin, Lee Rainie, and Monica Anderson, "53% of Americans Say the Internet Has Been Essential During the COVID-19 Outbreak," Pew Research Center, April 30, 2020, https://www.pewresearch.org.
2. "Internet/Broadband Fact Sheet," Pew Research Center, 2020, https://www.pewresearch.org.
3. "Labor Force Characteristics by Race and Ethnicity, 2018," U.S. Bureau of Labor Statistics, October 2019, https://www.bls.gov.
4. "Telehealth: Delivering Care Safely During COVID-19," U.S. Department of Health and Human Services, 2020, https://www.hhs.gov.
5. Reed Abelson, "Doctors and Patients Turn to Telemedicine in the Coronavirus Outbreak," *New York Times,* March 11, 2020, https://www.nytimes.com.
6. Jennifer Tolbert, Kendal Orgera, and Natalie Singer, "Key Facts about the Uninsured Population," Kaiser Family Foundation, December 13, 2019, https://www.kff.org.
7. "Health and Health Care for Blacks in the United States," Kaiser Family Foundation, May 10, 2019, https://www.kff.org.
8. "Health Equity Considerations and Racial and Ethnic Minority Groups," Centers for Disease Control and Prevention, July 24, 2020, https://www.cdc.gov.
9. Jayme Fraser and Dian Zhang, "The Poorest Will Suffer: Safety-Net Health Clinics Cut Services Amid Coronavirus Pandemic," *USA Today,* March 31, 2020, https://usatoday.com.
10. E. J. Dickson, "The Coronavirus Crisis in the Psychiatric Ward," *Rolling Stone,* April 13, 2020, https://www.rollingstone.com.
11. "KFF Health Tracking Poll—Early April 2020: The Impact of Coronavirus on Life in America," Kaiser Family Foundation, April 2, 2020, https://www.kff.org.
12. Jamie Smith Hopkins and Dean Russell, "The Mental Health Effects of Coronavirus Are a 'Slow-Motion Disaster,'" *Mother Jones,* April 2, 2020, https://www.motherjones.com.
13. Katharine Carter, "Working During COVID-19: Therapists Share Their Telemental Health Experiences," American Psychological Association, May 7, 2020, https://www.apa.org.
14. Matthew Perrone, "Virus Drives New Demand for Talkspace's Online Therapy," *Associated Press,* May 10, 2020, https://apnews.com; Anne Steel, "Pandemic, New Platforms Prompt Surge in New Therapists," *Wall Street Journal,* October 4, 2020, https://www.wsj.com; Katherine Ellison, "E-Therapy Apps See Booming Business Since Coronavirus Pandemic. I Gave One a Try," *Washington Post,* March 28, 2020, https://washingtonpost.com.

15. Jillian Mock, "Psychological Trauma Is the Next Crisis for Coronavirus Health Workers," *Scientific American,* June 1, 2020, https://www.scientificamerican.com.
16. Abdul Mannan Baig, "Neurological Manifestations in COVID-19 Caused by SARS-CoV-2," *CNS Neuroscience & Therapeutics* 26, no. 5 (2020): 499–501; Leonardo Jardim Vaz de Mello, Emylle Guimaraes Silva, Gabriel Oliveira Correa Rabelo, Mariana Evaristo Leite, Nathalia Ramos Vieira, Maryam Bahadori, Ali Seifi, and Daniel Agustin Godoy, "Neurologic Compromise in COVID-19: A Literature Review," *Journal of Neurology Research* 10, no. 5 (2020): 164–72.
17. The results of the study were shared on the CDC's website (https://www.cdc.gov/) although the study itself was published in a journal titled *Morbidity and Mortality Weekly Report.* See Mark É. Czeisler, Rashon I. Lane, Emiko Petrosky, Joshua F. Wiley, Aleta Christensen, Rashid Njai, Matthew D. Weaver, et al., "Mental Health, Substance Use, and Suicidal Ideation During the COVID-19 Pandemic—United States, June 24–30, 2020," *Morbidity and Mortality Weekly Report* 69, no. 32 (2020): 1053.
18. "SAMHSA Statement Regarding CDC's MMWR on Mental Health, Substance Use, and Suicidal Ideation During the COVID-19 Pandemic," Substance Abuse and Mental Health Services Administration, August 14, 2020, https://www.samhsa.gov.
19. "BLHF's COVID-19 Virtual Therapy—AVAILABLE NOW!," *Boris L. Henson Foundation,* 2020, https://borislhensonfoundation.org.
20. William Kole, "'Empire' Star Taraji P. Henson Hailed for Mental Health Work," *Washington Post,* October 8, 2020, https://www.washingtonpost.com.
21. Gwen Aviles, "Taraji P. Henson Creates Campaign to Offer African Americans Therapy During Pandemic," *NBC News,* April 16, 2020, https://www.nbcnews.com.
22. Jasmine Grant, "Exclusive: Taraji P. Henson Helps Those Affected by COVID-19 with Free Virtual Therapy," *Essence,* April 8, 2020, https://www.essence.co/.
23. Although screen-based therapy is an imperfect solution to an unmet demand for mental healthcare services, I believe it is currently much more important that persons in need of mental healthcare services receive them (even via teletherapy) than rule them out because of their delivery mechanism. Yet by extension, if we accept teletherapy, we must ensure adequate professional protections (including the ability to earn a living wage) for persons who work as teletherapists.

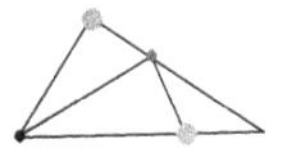

Index

Emma Bedor Hiland is a lecturer in the Department of Communication Studies at Texas Tech University.

Lightning Source UK Ltd.
Milton Keynes UK
UKHW020246110522
402785UK00003B/193